WELCOME!

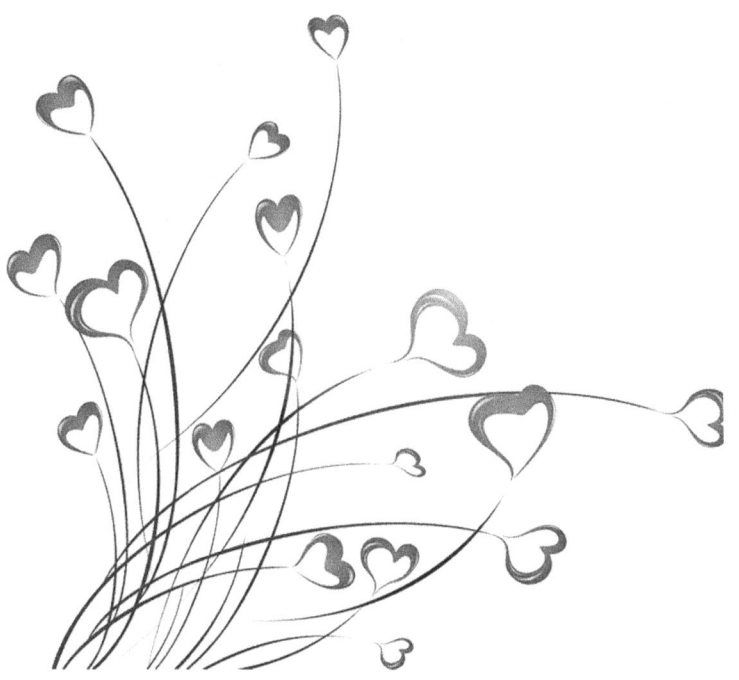

The author

Deirdre Boyd is CEO of the Addiction Recovery Foundation, editor of *Addiction Today*, and author of mental-health charity Mind's booklet *Understanding Addiction & Dependencies*. She is also founder and lead organiser of the UK/European Symposia on Addictive Disorders, the largest annual event devoted to recovery from addiction.

She is a member of the Centre for Policy Studies' Prisons and Addictions think-tank, of the Recovery Academy and of the Recovery Group. She participated in the dti's Office of Science & Technology project on *Brain Science, Addiction and Drugs*, forecasting the next two decades. She gave evidence on treatment for the government Select Committee on Cocaine 2010. She was also a trustee of the National Association for Children of Alcoholics UK.

In 2006, ICAA awarded her the Dr Vincent Bakeman memorial award for Outstanding Community Service In 2010, she was awarded a Sierra Tucson Pillar Of The Community award.

The author has practised all the addiction recovery techniques recommended in this book, which have kept her clean and sober since 1 July 1991.

♥   ♥   ♥

ADDICTIONS & RECOVERY: SELF-HELP FOR ADDICTS, FAMILIES, FRIENDS

BY DEIRDRE BOYD

♥ ♥ ♥

ADDICTIONS & RECOVERY: SELF-HELP FOR ADDICTS, FAMILIES, FRIENDS

Author, designer: Deirdre Boyd
Illustrations: Fotolia
(Indy's map in chapter 9 from Martin Weegmann)

ISBN: 1450562736
EAN-13: 978 1450562737
Version: 2.0

1st edition published by Element
as Addictions: Your questions answered
Copyright © Deirdre Boyd 1998-2010

A minimum 50% of royalties are donated to
The Addiction Recovery Foundation
charity no 328133

Contents

♥ ♥ ♥

Dedication and acknowledgments

This is both a dedication and acknowledgment to:

♥ the wonderful, dedicated team at the Addiction Recovery Foundation – Anthony Massouras, Ric Ohrstrom, Melissa Gordon, Suzanne Gooch for their almost-daily practical support, Dr Andrea Barthwell, Dave Mulvaney of Rapt, Hon David Bernstein, Steve Hamer, Kim Martin of Crossroads, Dave Mulvaney of Rapt, James Redpath of Mimosa, Kat Demeanour, Johan Sorensen

♥ the authors and publishers who gave permission to quote their works – read their pearls inside this book

♥ Molly Parkin and al kennedy for believing I had a book in me; and David Best, David Burrowes, Mary Brett, James Brokenshire, Huseyin Djemil, Gerald Deutsch, Professor Carlo DiClemente, Professor Carlton Erickson, Kathy Gyngell, Jim and Joan, Laurie Lipton, Benjamin (Lord) Mancroft, Professor Neil McKeganey, Laurence McMorrow, Niels Olsen, Steve Spiegel for their vital help

♥ My multitude of cousins especially Cha, Roisin and Clodagh; Bill Sharples and Uncle Liam; Rua, Buachaillin, Ruado; my much-loved brothers and sisters (Grainne, Sheila, Fiona, Dermot, Cormac, Shane, Aoife) – and *my father Harry and my mother Kitty.*

♥ ... And the many wonderful people who are committed to helping people recover – far too many to be able to list here, but we know who you are!

Forewords
1: Kathy Gyngell

"If there was ever a strong case to be made for extending awareness of the 12-Step programme, on which the advice in *Addictions & Recovery: Self-help for addicts, families, friends* is based, to everyone in society – and most of all to those in government responsible for spending the now billions allocated to drug treatment – the time for it is now.

For the message of this essential 'must keep by your side' guide to recovery and relapse risk is that addiction is a relative phenomenon from which no one is entirely immune. I defy anyone to assert, after reading the 'tests' set out on these pages, that none resonate, even though addiction might not have sent their lives spiralling out of control. How many of us, after all, can claim to be totally free from the deep psychological programming of negative early childhood experience that cuts across class and intelligence?

What also struck me reading this updated edition was that its insights and guidance, communicated with a clarity granted only to someone in recovery, are even more important than they were when they were first published. This is not because human nature is worse, nor simply because our increasingly liberal, highly individualistic and instant gratification culture creates an ever more fertile ground for social dysfunction and addiction. It is because there is a new factor in the equation to contend with.

This is the new level of intervention by the government in drugs treatment, under the auspices of the National Health Service, since Labour took office in 1997.

The period since then has seen unprecedented levels of government expenditure in 'treatment' – now running at nearly £1billion per annum – and a massive expansion of 'treatment services'. Yet far from achieving a recovery renaissance, this intervention has served only to entrench addiction. Services directed, not unreasonably, at the most problematic drug users rather than all who need help has not, sadly, been for the purpose of their recovery – they are routinely described in government documents as unrecoverable, abandoned by this self-fulfilling prophecy – but to reduce their crime.

Most shocking of all in this is the fact is that almost no government money has been allocated to supporting long-term problem users into either residential programmes linked to the 12 Steps or into counselling and peer-supported abstinence groups in the community. Research about their effectiveness has been ignored.

Instead, as fast as national prescribing and 'harm reduction' services have grown, previously government funded rehab beds have closed, as *Addiction Today* has systematically been documenting.

It seems that the policy architects who set the terms of the government's treatment programme from 1997 until this year fatally lacked the enlightenment and insights essential for successful addiction treatment, which could have easily been drawn from those who have successfully recovered, the vast majority through 12-Step principles.

Any realistic treatment policy must be based on the following simple truths.

- If you cannot get the drug you love, you get the drug you are near (policy application: addiction is not substance or behaviour specific but must be addressed in its totality)
- Family members who try to manage, restrain or control 'their' addict's behaviour are fighting a losing battle and can be complicit as families in denial and/or actively codependent (policy application: the state risks adopting the role of codependent by 'managing' addicts through prescription; it risks sponsoring addiction)
- The 'healthy' family response is to stop conspiring with dependency behaviour or being party to it (policy applcation: the state must not collude with depending behaviour – rather confront it where it harms and risks others, yet fully support the addict motivated for recovery)
- The illusion of control over addiction which addicts insist they have is just that, an illusion (policy application: the state must not be manipulated by persuasive addictive behaviour and demands, addicts should not decide their dosage).

Instead we have a treatment policy which bizarrely excludes alcohol and one in which clinicians doom patient to never being 'ready for recovery' – because they misconstrue addictive behaviour.

As 2010 decade opens, government policy has put today's drug addict in a new and harder place, not just up against addiction but up against the state, too. It puts those with a primary alcohol addiction as before, bereft of the funding for rehab interventions which work and even less chance of medically supervised inpatient detox followed directly by entry to rehab.

So never was there more need for the self-help tactics and peer support which Deirdre Boyd sets out so logically, honestly and compassionately in her book, nor for the widest possible dissemination of these messages.

In fact, with the first sign of official dismay at the scale of waste and dysfunction of the government's policy to date – one which sees no more people in recovery than would be without it, and the Home Office kept in the dark about its impact – witnessed in the recently published Public Accounts Committee censure, and with an election this year, the updated reprint of *Addictions & Recovery: Self-help for addicts, families, friends* could not be more timely. **"**

♥ ♥ ♥

Kathy Gyngell is research fellow at the Centre for Policy Studies and chair of its Prisons and Addictions Forum. She has chaired and authored two *Addictions* volumes for *Breakdown Britain* and *Breakthrough Britain*, the Social Justice Policy Review for the Conservative Party.

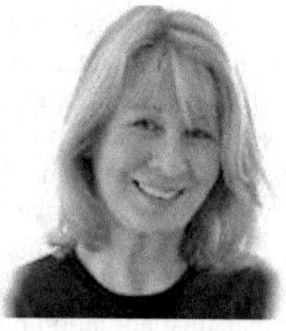

Forewords
2. David Best

"In the past few years, there has been justifiable excitement at the emergence of a UK recovery movement which continues to gather energy, dynamism and confidence. However, this should not mask the fact that recovery is not something new – and that Britain is replete with rich and varied success stories, and an incredible wealth of the recovery wisdom and insight that courses through Deirdre's book.

This book is an important chapter in an unfolding narrative that combines a critical approach to the clinical hegemony which has dominated the ownership of knowledge, and rightly sheds a light on the incredible stories of success and recovery that supersede the much more pallid and flaccid goals of formalised 'treatment'.

Thus the focus on key decisions about families and relationships, about jobs and opportunities and the basic survival skills required for a recovery journey provide the lived experience of recovery and the core for both giving something back and, for readers, the opportunity to learn the lived-experience of their recovery as it occurs in real settings outside a clinic.

Our knowledge of the mechanisms and catalysts for addiction recovery are at an early stage – there is still much for us to understand and observe about the processes of individual, family and community recovery – so this book is a significant contribution from an important voice.

The body of recovery literature will have some of the key qualities of recovery itself: a celebration of hope and belief, a celebration of perseverance and commitment, and a diversity of events and pathways that are shared as part of the mutuality of helping and being helped.

Recovery is a miraculous story and this book provides an insight into some everyday miracles and replicable successes. 🙰

♥ ♥ ♥

Dr David Best is reader in criminal justice at the University of Western Scotland. He was senior lecturer in addictions in the department of psychiatry at Birmingham University, spent 10 years in research at the National Addiction Centre/Institute of Psychiatry in London, including 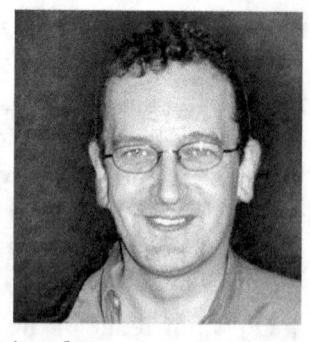 secondments to the National Treatment Agency and Prime Minister's Delivery Unit.

Forewords
3: Prof Neil McKeganey

"Deirdre Boyd's book is being updated at a crucial time. There is more interest now in recovery than there has been for the last 30 years. Indeed, over that time the very notion of recovery has been little more than a sideline to a drugs treatment industry driven by the philosophy of harm reduction. Interest now is returning to the issue of how treatment services can actually help individuals to recover from their dependency.

In Scotland, for the first time we have a drug strategy which defines recovery in terms of enabling drug users to become drug free. In England, too, our politicians are beginning to realise that drug treatment services need to be about more than enabling people to 'manage' their ongoing addiction.

If the world of professional drug treatment turned its face away from the notion of recovery, the 12-Step self-help movement never did.

Those who have undergone recovery know more than anyone else the true power of people with dependency committing themselves to helping each other. Deirdre's book is full of the wisdom of personal experience of recovery and is written with a journalist's ease of communication. Read this book to find out about the techniques of recovery that can guide you in the dark moments of your addiction. Read this book to recognise that in the journey of recovery, who you are, and what you have been, is not the same as who you can become.

This is a book that is run through with a wisdom borne of personal experience. As the drugs treatment industry belatedly takes up the challenge of recovery, it needs to rapidly acquire the knowledge, hard won, of those who never lost sight of what it means to confront one's addiction and move on.

In the US, there are doctors who prescribe 12-Step recovery to their addicted patients. In the UK, there are doctors who find it hard to see beyond the next page on their prescription pad. I hope that this book plays its part in changing that culture and making abstinence-based recovery the goal of treatment. **"**

♥ ♥ ♥

Professor Neil McKeganey is professor of Drug Misuse Research and founding director of the Centre for Drug Misuse Research, University of Glasgow. He has advised the UK Home Office, the World Health Organisation and the US Department of Justice.

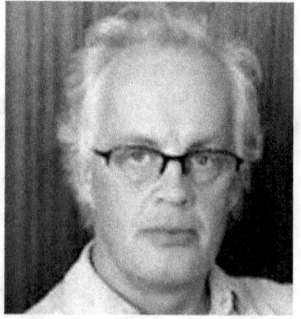

Introduction

> **"** Just for today, I will allow myself to be as happy as I want to be. **"** Excerpt from AA's *Just For Today* card

Addiction is probably the only illness which you must understand in order to recover from it. By the time you have finished this book, you will certainly have that understanding – in fact, as it contains up-to-date information from the best sources that I can find in my professional capacity as editor of the only UK magazine devoted to recovery, *Addiction Today*, you will have as much information as many professionals in the field.

Sufferers, their families and friends – often including the highly intelligent and the highly educated – usually feel powerless to stop the damage done by and to an addict, and look on helplessly. The aim of this book is to help understand what is happening, to take away that feeling of powerlessness and to guide both sufferer and those close to him or her towards a life of help, support and peace of mind.

Chapter 1 identifies features which are common to all addictions. These similarities highlight the fact that you can also find similarities in solutions and sources of help.

Chapter 2 follows this with check-lists of symptoms for specific kinds of addiction, both chemical (ie, alcohol and drugs) and non-chemical (ie, behaviours such as bingeing, working, shopping or gambling), and for obsessive-compulsive disorders.

Chapter 3 looks at the 'causes' of addiction. Ground-breaking research emerging only since the 1990s shows that both substance and behavioural addictions are linked to pre-existing chemical imbalances in the body. Potential addicts ineffectively process "feelgood" chemicals which circulate naturally in other people's bodies. They can only "feelgood" by using an artificial substance which replaces these chemicals' actions – but simultaneously sets up the addictive process. Learning how this chemical chain works can help us to understand that stopping has nothing to do with intelligence or will power – only with not taking that first drink, drug or other object of addiction which sets up the chemical chain.

Low levels of "feelgood" chemicals can be further depleted by pivotal childhood events. By tracing their origin, we can put them in context and react to them in a positive way which raises the levels naturally.

Chapter 4 details self-help tactics for emergencies when you feel you must use your addiction. Chapter 5 shows how to use "boundaries" – invisible physical and emotional shields – to protect you while learning both these tactics and the longer-term strategies described in Chapter 6. They are worth practising when professional therapists are not available, between therapy sessions even when you have a therapist, between self-help meetings, and to see how much you can improve things by yourself.

If there is a '12-Step' group for your particular addiction, you might not need to seek professional help as it will support your self-management and suggest even more ways of recovery. Chapter 7 explains 12-Step groups.

If, despite all of these, you find that you still cannot stop your addiction, it is time to seek professional help. Chapter 8 examines first of all some ways in which people close to an addict might persuade them to accept help to change. Chapter 9 then explaines the different types of treatment available: individual, group, daycare and residential. It also explains what to look for in your treatment provider, and what you might expect in the course of therapy.

Chapter 10 deals with the special case of adolescents. Most teenagers will not have lived long enough to have committed often enough the highly shaming, damaging actions which older adults have gone through in the course of their addiction, and which forced them to seek help. Teenagers also follow their peers rather than older adults, even though the former may be drinking and drugging and the latter clean and sober. However, we can open their eyes and minds to the value of life without addiction.

Offenders in the courts and criminal justice system are also reluctant to enter treatment. One of the adolescents' programmes can work for them, too.

Chapter 11 deals with the special cases of 'dual disorders': another disorder accompanying the addiction and which might have been masked by it. The most common are depression, personality disorders and schizophrenia. It is vital that these cases are diagnosed as relapse from one disorder will lead to relapse into the other. Dual disorder must mean dual recovery.

This chapter also deals with an often-neglected minority: people with physical disabilities. Carers often mistakenly think that they are an exception, that their addiction is all disabled people have to make a hard life easier. But the addiction is the most crippling disability of all and must be tackled in order to improve quality of life.

DEFINITIONS OF RECOVERY

> " Recovery is a process through which an individual is enabled to move-on from their problem drug use towards a drug-free life and become an active and contributing member of society "
>
> Scottish government drug policy document 2008: The Road To Recovery.

> " Recovery from substance dependence is a voluntarily maintained lifestyle characterised by sobriety, personal health and citizenship "
>
> Betty Ford Institute Consensus Panel, 2007

The US government's drug policy this year gives a similar definition but adds "... with or without medication".

♥ ♥ ♥

I would be delighted to hear from readers who have found this book helpful.
You can contact me c/o
The Addiction recovery Foundation
193 Victoria Street
London SW1E 5NE
info@addictiontoday.org

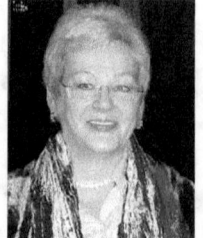

1

What addictions have in common

" *I held a high-profile job with a multinational company. I owned my own house. I was in a seven-year relationship. To an observer, I looked as though I had it all. But I was miserable....*

What my family didn't know was that I had started drinking in the office, risking my job. I was in arrears with my mortgage. Despite my good salary, I couldn't pay the bills. My boyfriend was becoming violent and insulting me and I was trying more and more to please him. People stopped inviting me to social events. "

Catherine

" *I grew up thinking that workaholism was a virtue. I turned down social engagements because I 'had to' work. I missed family events because I 'had to' work – it was the only excuse my workaholic family understood and accepted. In the end, I couldn't have a conversation unless it was about work. I socialised only with work colleagues. In 17 years of working, I took only three weeks' holiday. By my late 30s, I was lonely. I did not earn as much as counterparts who worked far less. I feared that if I asked for a pay rise I might lose my job. I was like an alcoholic who was being paid to drink – there was no way I would question the payment.* "

John

Sometimes there is just a hint or two of addiction, that something is not quite right, unsettling. It becomes far more painful later, both for someone desperate to stop but cannot, and for those helplessly watching a friend, colleague, loved one or family member sink into the degradation which accompanies full-blown addiction.

The true situations described by Catherine and John on the previous page show journeys from one to the other.

On the way, there will have been increasing suffering from shame, rages, arguments, financial difficulties, social embarrassments, stress, unpredictability, accidents and injuries, and emotional and physical illnesses. Usually, too, there will have been job losses and loss of relationships.

The good news is: there are solutions which work. And you do not have to reach the worst stages of addiction, the so-called "rock bottom", before you try them to halt then improve your situation. You can follow these solutions by yourself and with others.

This chapter looks at what is common to all addictions. It also gives a check-list for "codependency" which is not only a dependency in itself – to people or substances – but also accompanies every other addiction. Recovery from codependency is part of recovery from any addiction.

Chapter 2 gives check-lists for the most common types of addiction: to alcohol, drugs, bingeing on food, starving, work, sex, love, gambling, shopping, religion and other compulsive behaviours. Because of all the commonalities, there are common solutions, described in Chapter 4.

♥ ♥ ♥

First of all, a definition of what addiction is *not*.
It is nothing to do with lack of willpower or intelligence.
In fact, if you are an addict in recovery, you probably
have above-normal willpower and intelligence.

A recent definition of addiction by neuro (brain) scientists is that it is a "dysregulation of the mesolimbic dopamine system" – but more of that in chapter 3, which looks at the 'causes' of addiction. The point is that we are dealing with an illness that can be put in remission.

THE PARADOX OF ADDICTION

Addiction is probably the only disorder in the world which you must understand in order to recover from it. It involves many paradoxes. For example, whether you are addicted to a "substance" or to a behaviour, you are looking for an escape from pain of which you might no longer be aware, or from memories which you might no longer consciously remember.

Addicts have low self-esteem yet can appear arrogant, with a "superfiority" complex. They can hate themselves, even though they can present a successful mask to the world (and gamblers can feel a sense of overconfidence, power and control). They often feel ashamed, and that they deserve to be punished. They can be lonely, perhaps especially so when surrounded by friends.

They can feel that their world is falling apart and they have no control over it – yet some hold high-functioning jobs or appear all-controlling to the people around them.

If you are an addict, you have probably already noticed that you are overly concerned with the approval of others and are sensitive to criticism. Despite your downward spiral, you are usually a perfectionist.

Most addicts are cut off – dissociated – from their feelings and their bodies, so much so that they don't even know it. When an addict is asked how he or she feels, they inevitably start their reply with "I think...". The reaction comes from the intellect, not the body. For instance, have you scared people with your rage, then denied you were angry – and meant it? When someone has commented that you looked sad, have you denied the evidence of their eyes, and believed that you told the truth?

Sadly, addicts are not cut off from every feeling. If you are reading this book, you will have felt the most intense: fear, shame, loneliness, desperation and increasing despair that you cannot change how things are. The only euphoric feeling has probably come from excitement, an adrenalin buzz. This is why the search for excitement can be both an addiction in itself and reinforce other addictions – such as shoplifting giving a buzz as well as funding drugs. It also explains politicians, sports stars and others having affairs not *despite* but *because* they threaten things they hold dear in their lives.

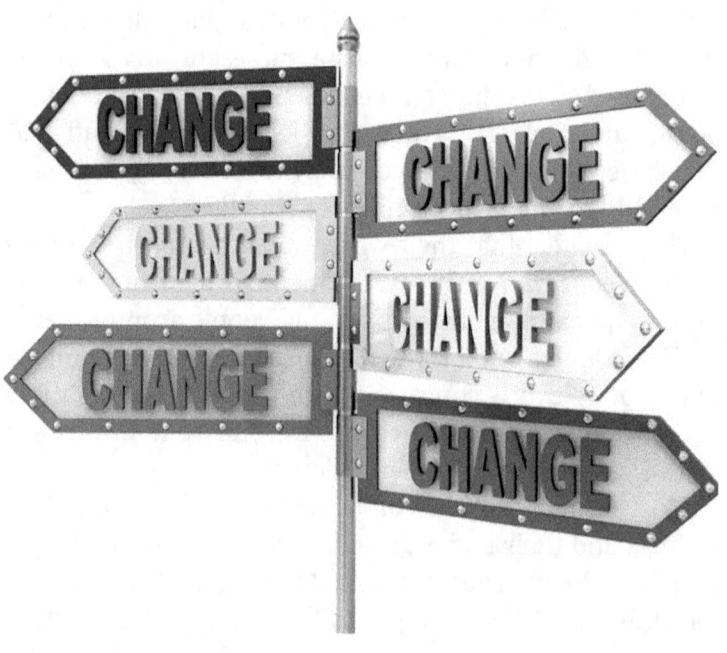

WHAT IS COMMON TO ALL ADDICTIONS

All addicts need more and more of their addiction to achieve the same level of initial euphoria or intoxication; you get less and less satisfaction from the same 'volume' of addiction. This symptom is known as increased "tolerance".

Almost every addict has tried to control, reduce or stop using but has managed to succeed for limited periods only, if at all, despite best intentions and efforts. This is another recognised symptom.

Addicts' thoughts are preoccupied with their substance or behaviour. You can spend large chunks of time not only "using" (ie, using your addiction) but also thinking about using or giving it up, trying to fund the addiction, getting into activities which help you to use, and trying to make up for the consequences of a bad bout of using.

Addicts are drawn to acquaintances of similar habits, so that their own behaviour does not look too bad in comparison with them.

You, or someone close to you, might also have jeopardised or lost close relationships, educational opportunities and jobs. You or they might have engaged in "bailout" behaviour, turning to family or others for help with financial or other problems – but not the addiction itself.

You or they might have asserted something on the lines of "If you had my problems, you would drink/drug/use, too". This is called denial; after all, it is the addictive behaviours which cause and intensify problems.

An outside observer will notice a pattern to addiction: preoccupation, denial, craving and relapse back into the addiction and its accompanying behaviour, all getting progressively worse.

Internally, I believe that one vital ingredient in addiction is a grief which was not allowed to be expressed in childhood so that it intensified, ignored, over decades. This grief can be from emotional, physical or sexual abuse or the loss of a loved one through death, divorce or separation. Tracing the source and grieving in recovery is a predictor of good progress.

In reading this chapter, it might become obvious that addicts have neurotic behaviour. In one sense, this gives hope, as neurotics tend to be over-responsible, which can be turned into an asset: neurotic people tend to take responsibility for their recovery, once started.

You might be ashamed to tell anyone about your problem – but if you do not, and you do not hear of others with similar or worse problems, how can you hear about solutions? They are found in the experiences of others who have been through what you are going through.

CODEPENDENCY

I have never known an addict who was not also codependent. Codependency – the "in" word of the 1980s, then ignored through complacency and now returning to attention – is the addiction to 'looking elsewhere'. This can include substances or behaviours but is mainly taken to mean codependency on other people, looking to them rather than ourselves for happiness and fulfilment.

It goes hand in hand with addiction and can lead to relapse into other addictions.

That is why it is so vital to learn about 'boundaries' – see chapter 5 – and create healthy relationships. As well as giving satisfaction and a new world of benefits, they help to prevent relapse back into the addiction and despair.

There is a joke which defines it well: "A codependent is someone who finds out how you are before they can tell you how they are". Another descriptive joke is that "When a codependent is about to die, someone else's life flashes before their eyes".

In other words, if you are codependent, people's reactions matter so much to you that, if you cannot handle them, you can turn to addiction instead. How to handle your reaction to other people is learned through the "boundaries" explained in Chapter 5.

Codependents act as though they have extra-sensory perception. In other words, you guess what other people are feeling or might feel towards a particular situation, then you alter all your actions around that potential reaction so as "not to upset anyone". But you do not ask and discover anyone's true feelings in the first place, so often end up with the very reaction you do not want.

You can also inadvertently irritate people because they cannot sense what you want or need. One small example: have you ever felt disappointed because people give you birthday presents which indicate they cannot tell what would please you? But perhaps you expect them to know without ever having expressed to them what makes you happy – because you don't know yourself.

Codependents cannot express their wants and needs because they do not know what they are, being in the habit of subjugating them to others. This can lead to mental and physical exhaustion and illnesses.

Extreme dependence – emotionally, socially and sometimes physically – on another person or object affects all other relationships. In *Co-Dependence: Healing The Human Condition*, Dr Charles Whitfield sees it as a personality disorder based on a need to control despite adverse results, neglecting your own needs, intense pain through intimacy/separation, getting involved with people who are not good for you, and other signs such as "denial, constricted feelings, depression and stress-related medical illness".

You can become addicted not only to people who are close to your heart but even to people you do not like, such as a nuisance neighbour. You can become as preoccupied with that bad neighbour and their hostile actions as a love addict is with their partner. Al-Anon for friends and families of alcoholics can be helpful with this.

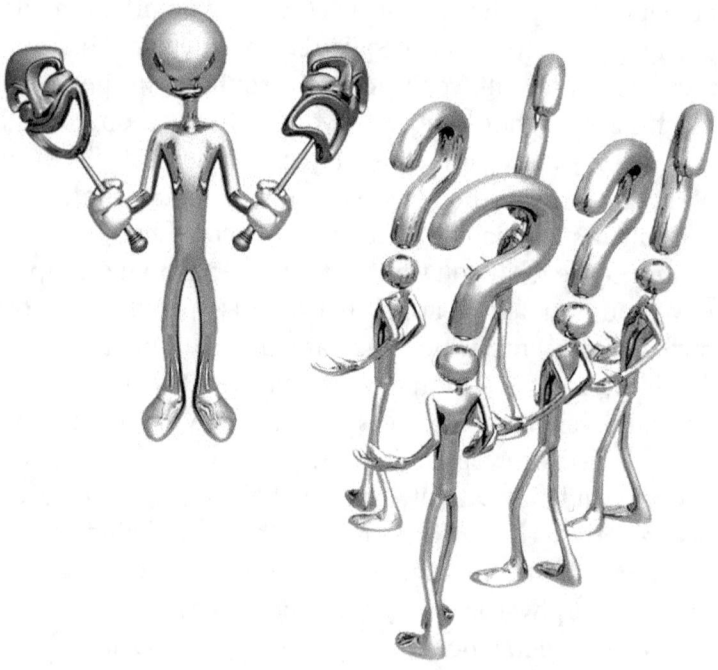

On the next page are some of the 31 questions Dr Whitfield uses to diagnose codependency (see more questions on codependent relationships in Chapter 6).

ARE YOU CODEPENDENT?

1. *Do you seek approval and affirmation?*
2. *Do you fail to recognise your accomplishments?*
3. *Do you fear criticism?*
4. *Do you have a need for perfection?*
5. *Are you uneasy when your life is going smoothly? Do you continually anticipate problems?*
6. *Do you care for others easily, but find it hard to care for yourself?*
7. *Do you attract/seek people who tend to be compulsive?*
8. *Do you cling to relationships?*
9. *Is it hard for you to relax and have fun?*
10. *Do you have an over-developed sense of responsibility?*
11. *Do you have a tendency to chronic fatigue, aches and pains?*
12. *Do you have difficulty asking for what you want from others?*

Codependency can leave you feeling so empty that you try to fill that emptiness in unhealthy ways which lead to emotional and physical illness, including "self medicating". Again, the solution comes from using "boundaries", introduced in Chapter 5.

ADDICTIVE SOCIETY

We are an addictive society. Everyone will feel some of the symptoms described in this and the following chapter to some degree. It does not necessarily mean that you are addicted: it is to what degree it affects your life that is important.

Recovering from addiction means a new and fulfilling way of life, a happier and healthier one. The trials of everyday life must still be dealt with, but our attitude to them can change: crises can happen around us, not *to* us.

If this can be achieved by addicts who were once spiralling to destruction, it can offer hope and lessons for family members also.

♥　♥　♥

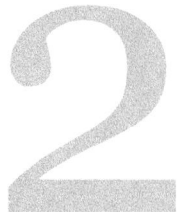

Check-lists for addictions

" I met Peter while on holiday abroad and we had a wonderful time. He had a great body, although I did wonder how preoccupied he might be with bodybuilding. He also ate and drank a lot but he said that he rarely did so at home; this was a holiday.

When he invited me round to his place two weeks later, we bumped into a pal who greeted him with the words "Nice to see you sober for once". I don't want to get into a relationship with someone who has a drink or food problem. I know it will all turn sour. But I do want him. Is he really addicted? **"**

Robin

" I noticed Anne at lunch because she was hiding a slice of brown bread under her hand, sliding it off the table onto her lap. When she left, she was still hiding it. It was very peculiar because she could just have eaten it openly, like everyone else at the table.

A few nights later, I switched on the kitchen light and found that she had been standing in the dark, rooting in the food cupboards. It's not as though she was stealing a lot of food, and she did have a right to it, anyway. I just couldn't understand why she was taking it like a thief. She looked so guilty at being caught. **"**

Patricia

How can you know if someone close to you is addicted? Sometimes it is painfully clear, such as with the girl injecting in the left of the photo below. Other times, such as with the ill-looking girl on the right, it is questionable if someone is acting addictively, even if the harm seems obvious: "I can stop any time I want" is a common defence.

If you want to learn, or perhaps you want written proof with a list of symptoms, this chapter gives check-lists

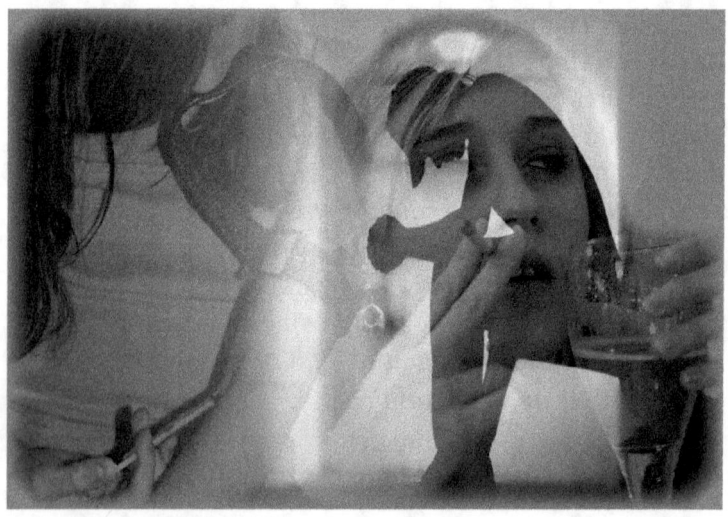

of symptoms for specific addictions. Some are medical criteria, others have been compiled by specialists in their fields with decades of experience and/or by self-help groups. These can confirm whether you need to take action, or not.

You can also show them to the person you are concerned about; you might not get any immediate reaction – you might even be met with anger – but you will have sown the seed of recovery. People believe what they see written in black and white far more than something they hear.

Perhaps you think you have a problem and you have already decided to do something about it. In that case, I hope that the check-lists will reassure you that you are not alone, that you are neither "mad" nor "bad" but similar to a lot of other people, and that you can recover from the illness as others with these symptoms have done.

How do we define substance dependence or addiction? For the purposes of this book, we shall use "addiction" as the all-embracing description accepted by most of the general public. I also see this as interchangeable with "dependence". Addiction/dependence is very different from abusing/misusing drugs, although they often appear similar to the observer – this chapter will list the symptoms of both, for greatest clarity.

It is worth knowing that even professionals working in the treatment field do not always agree on the terminology, that therapists and neuroscientists use addiction/ dependence interchangeably – but doctors can use them with different meanings. Developments in government drug policies could lead to the definition used in this book becoming the common standard.

In the meantime, "dependency" is used as often as "dependence", and "chemical" as often as "substance". Some professionals also define addiction as applying only to a mood-altering chemical/drug/substance and dependency as applying to behaviours to achieve the same effect, such as gambling or workaholism. Still others prefer "dependence" to differentiate between emotional dependence only or physically dependence addressed merely by 'detox'. And others argue as to whether they prefer the word "abuse" or "misuse".

If talking with professionals, you might want to clarify that you are using the official definitions in this chapter.

DEFINITIONS OF ADDICTION/DEPENDENCE

"Probably the best way to see alcoholism or drug addiction is as a progressive fatal disease with established genetic and brain-chemical factors, and is seen in behaviours such as loss of control over drinking/drugging, denial and craving," states Dr Michael Wilks of the Medical Council on Alcoholism in London and currently president of the Standing Committee of European Doctors.

The two most widely used definitions of addiction/dependence, with accompanying lists of symptoms, come from the World Health Organisation and the American Psychiatric Association.

The World Health Organisation's *ICD-10 International Classification of Diseases-10th revision*, printed in 2004, defines "the dependence syndrome" as "physiological, behavioural and cognitive phenomena in which the use of a substance or class of substances takes on a much higher priority for a given individual than other behaviours that once had greater value... central is the desire to take psychoactive drugs (which may or not have been medically prescribed), alcohol or tobacco".

In 1994, the American Psychiatric Association published a definition in its *DSM-IV Diagnostic & Statistical Manual*, under the heading of substance dependence (the updated *DSM-V* is due in 1012). The *DSM-IV* calls it a group of mental, physical and behaviour symptoms showing "continued use of the substance despite significant substance-related problems. There is a pattern of repeated self-administration that usually results in tolerance, withdrawal and compulsive drug-taking behaviour."

Most of this is obvious, but 'tolerance' and 'withdrawal' might require explanation. First, let me reassure that, although it sounds daunting, you can send alcohol and drug addiction into lifelong remission. "It is the only disease which can be cured by talking," many recoverers state (see Chapters 4, 6 and 7).

SYMPTOMS: TOLERANCE AND WITHDRAWAL

Tolerance is either a need for markedly increased amounts of the substance to achieve intoxification/desired effect, or a markedly reduced effect despite continued use of the same amount. Many addicts find the latter frightening and try even more of the substance to achieve the same glorious effects they initially felt. When this no longer works – a stage for which you can wait 10 years – you can get such a shock that you try recovery.

Withdrawal signs can develop within hours or days after stopping or reducing substance use – many people are familiar with the phrase "cold turkey" to describe heroin withdrawal without medication. Withdrawal from the heroin substitute methadone is even more painful.

If you have tried to withdraw from alcohol, you might have suffered sweating, high pulse rate, hand tremors, insomnia, nausea or vomiting, hallucinations, anxiety or fits. Alcohol can be the most lethal of all drugs to quit suddenly if you have been overdrinking, so you might need professional help. If your doctor cannot or will not help, many rehabs have their own 'detox' facility to get you started on the road to recovery. The bonus of a rehab is that it will support you after detox.

Withdrawal from amphetamine/cocaine includes dysphoria (opposite of euphoria), fatigue, unpleasant dreams, insomnia or hypersomnia, increased appetite and slowed or agitated reactions.

Withdrawal from opioids – morphine, heroin, codeine, methadone, even diarrheal agents and cough suppressants – includes dysphoria, nausea or vomiting, muscle aches, crying or running nose, pupillary dilation, goose pimples or sweating, diarrhoea, yawning, fever and insomnia.

Nicotine withdrawal is easy to recognise. It includes depression, insomnia, irritability, frustration or anger, anxiety, difficulty concentrating, restlessness, decreased heart rate and increased appetite.

Caffeine withdrawal includes fatigue or drowsiness, anxiety or depression and nausea or vomiting.

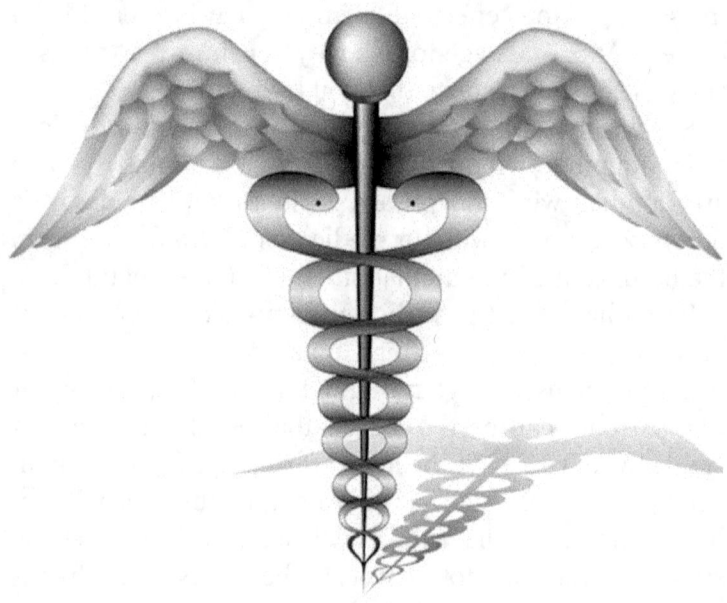

Most addicts today are 'polydrug' users, proving how easy it is to become 'cross addicted' and emphasising that destructive behaviours will continue if only one drug is treated rather than common causes.

SYMPTOMS FOR SUBSTANCE DEPENDENCE

1. Tolerance (increased amounts/reduced effects)
2. Withdrawal syndrome, or using another substance to avoid withdrawal symptoms
3. Often using larger amounts or using for longer periods than intended
4. A persistent desire or unsuccessful efforts to cut down or control substance use
5. Spending much time obtaining the substance – for example, visiting multiple doctors or off-licences, driving long distances
6. Giving up or reducing important social, occupational or recreational activities because of substance use
7. Continuing substance use despite knowing you have a persistent or recurrent physical or psychological problem likely to have been caused or exacerbated by the substance – for example, using cocaine despite getting cocaine-induced depression or drinking despite knowing that it is making your ulcer worse.

If items 1 and 2 are not present, there is no physical dependence [yet].

DSM-IV, American Psychiatric Association

The *ICD-10* confirms that a "definite diagnosis" of dependence should usually be made if three or more of the following were present together at some time during the previous year:

✓ Strong desire or sense of compulsion to take the substance
✓ Difficulties in controlling substance-taking behaviour in terms of its onset, termination or levels of use
✓ A physiological withdrawal state when substance use

has ceased or reduced, evidenced by characteristic withdrawal syndrome for the substance or use of the same (or closely related) substance with the intention of relieving or avoiding withdrawal symptoms

✓ Evidence of tolerance – increased doses of the psychoactive substance are required to achieve effects originally produced by lower doses

✓ Progressive neglect of alternative pleasures or interests because of psychoactive substance use, increased time to obtain/take the substance or recover from its effects

✓ Persisting with substance use despite clear evidence of overtly harmful consequences, such as harm to the liver through excessive drinking, depression after heavy substance use, or drug-related impairment of cognitive functioning.

SYMPTOMS FOR SUBSTANCE ABUSE

Some people can abuse substances without being dependent – they can stop or cut back if they wish. But, during a 12-month period they will show, like addicts, one or more of these signs of clinically significant distress:

1. Recurrent substance use results in a failure to fulfill major obligations at work, school or home – for example, absenteeism, poor work performance, suspensions or expulsions from school, neglect of children or home

1. Substance is used in physically hazardous situations – for example, drink-driving or operating a machine.

DSM-IV

The ICD-10 refers to "harmful use" rather than abuse, and states that "harmful use should not be diagnosed if dependence syndrome... is present".

FOOD

Almost every one of the women I know who have exceptionally good figures suffer from a food disorder and continuously think themselves too fat. In my experience, people who are "very average" or "mildly plump" are happier with their imperfect figures than food addicts are with their near-perfect ones.

Sadly, with the growing pressure by society for super-thin super-model figures, studies have discovered a significant number of children as young as six to be worried about their body image.

Food addictions are generally divided into two types: anorexia nervosa and bulimia nervosa. There are also overeaters, who differ in that they see themselves as smaller than they are whereas anorexics and bulimics see themselves at least 30% larger than they actually are.

Anorexics usually starve themselves, although a few also binge and purge like bulimics. Adults with anorexia have been admitted to hospital weighing as little as four stone – seeing themselves as overweight all the way there. But the most life-threatening eating disorder is suffered by people who swing between anorexia and bulimia, because the strain on the body from the effects of starving then bingeing and purging is so great.

If you are anorexic, you might have tried to hide your behaviour by saying that you are becoming vegan or obsessively searching out health-food shops. You might have exercised addictively to lose weight or, in the USA particularly, become addicted to "cut and tuck" – plastic surgery, liposuction, etc.

SYMPTOMS FOR ANOREXIA NERVOSA

The most widely-used definitions of anorexia are found in the *DSM-IV* and *ICD-10*. The *DSM-IV* list is below.
1. Refusal to maintain body weight at/above a minimal normal weight for age and height – body weight is usually less than 85% of the expected weight
2. Intense fear of gaining weight or becoming fat, even though underweight
3. Disturbance in body image – sufferer sees all or a part of the body as fat, even though underweight
4. In women, absence of at least three consecutive menstrual cycles.

The following are also characteristics of anorexia: hair loss, dry skin, brittle nails, insomnia, low blood pressure, low body temperature and heart rate, feeling cold/poor circulation and lanugo growth – fine hair growing all over the body, including the face.

The *ICD-10* criteria are similar, but in addition, specifically mention the ways in which people might induce weight-loss or maintain low body weight (avoiding fattening foods, self-induced vomiting, self-induced purging, excessive exercise, excessive use of appetite suppressants or diuretics).

ICD-10 also mentions physiological features: "widespread endocrine disorder involving hypothalamic-pituitary-gonadal axis is manifest in women as amenorrhoea and in men as loss of sexual interest and potency. There may also be elevated levels of growth hormones, raised cortisol levels, changes in the peripheral metabolism of thyroid hormone and abnormalities of insulin secretion".

In other words, if anorexia starts before puberty, that development is delayed or arrested. Semistarvation as an anorexic can affect most of your body organs, as can your use of laxatives, diuretics and enemas. Anaemia is a common side-effect.

SYMPTOMS FOR BULIMIA NERVOSA

If you are a bulimic, you will have indulged in binge eating and compensatory purging to prevent weight gain, and done this at least twice a week on average for three months. You will also have tried to eat in secrecy (see Anne's story on the first page of this chapter).

You might plan an eating binge in advance and not stop until you are painfully full. You might then feel a lack of control, and self-hatred. This is worse than anorexia in that you can feel that you are a "failed anorexic".

The *DSM-IV* defines bulimia nervosa as below.

1. Recurrent binge eating – ie, eating in a specific period of time (such as any two hours) more food than most people would eat in a similar time and circumstance – with a sense of lack of control over eating

2. Recurrent inappropriate compensatory behaviour to prevent weight gain, such as vomiting; misuse of laxatives, diuretics, enemas or other medications; fasting; or excessive exercise

3. Both the above occur, on average, at least twice a week for three months
4. Self-evaluation is unduly influenced by body shape and weight.

The *ICD-10* describes bulimia nervosa as characterised by repeated overeating and an excessive preoccupation with the control of body weight, leading to a pattern of overeating followed by vomiting or use of purgatives.

"This disorder shares many psychological features with anorexia nervosa, including an overconcern with body shape and weight," it reveal. "Repeated vomiting is likely to give rise to disturbances of body electrolytes and physical complications. There is often, but not always, a history of an earlier episode of anorexia nervosa."

You can damage your tooth enamel as a result of persistent vomiting, and get bad breath, digestive disorders and irritation of your throat and mouth.

OVEREATING

Just as there are people who abuse mood-altering substances but are not addicted, there are people who "comfort eat" or compulsively overeat. The *DSM-IV* does not give a list of symptoms but Chambers Concise 20th Century Dictionary defines it as "a strong irrational, constant and irresistible impulse to eat too much" while *ICD-10* refers to "overeating due to stressful events, such as bereavement, accident, childbirth, etc".

Unlike bulimics, comfort eaters do not usually compensate by over-exercising, vomiting or taking laxatives. They are thus more noticeable by their large size.

Although not mentioned in *DSM-IV* or *ICD-10*, it is my belief that much overeating – especially in recovering alcoholics – could be due to sugar imbalances. For women, this can be most pronounced during "that time of the month" when blood:sugar levels swing wildly, or during peri/menopause.

♥ ♥ ♥

The first step in recovering from food addictions and comfort eating is to avoid so-called "trigger foods". These are usually reminiscent of childhood treats and usually refined-sugar-based or dairy produce like cream and cheese; they can trigger you into bingeing on almost anything. Avoidance of trigger foods can be reinforced with a healthy diet – more research is emerging as to what foods can help rebalance your body chemistry in recovery – and with the suggestions in this book.

With bulimia, an important step is also to avoid the 'rituals' which can lead into bingeing/vomiting/purging.

Finally: "chocoholism". There have been claims that chocolate, or cocoa, releases chemicals in the brain similar to those experienced when smoking marijuana. But recent scientific opinion is that there is little in cocoa to make it addictive and that "chocoholics" are, in fact, conditioned by the food's sweet taste and fatty texture.

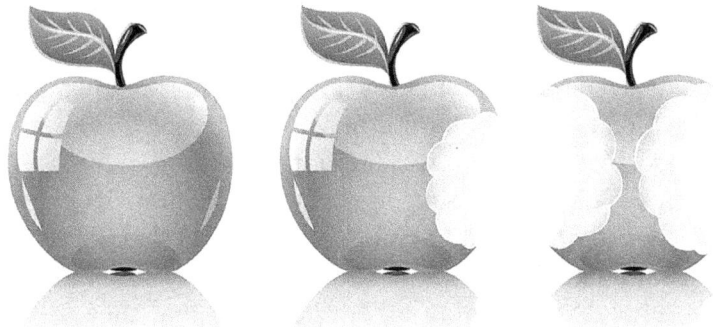

SYMPTOMS FOR ADDICTIVE GAMBLING

Addictive gambling is persistent and disrupts personal, family or vocational pursuits. Most gamblers say that they are seeking "action" – euphoria or an adrenalin buzz – more than money.

Gambling mirrors chemical addiction in that increasingly larger bets or greater risks might be needed to produce the desired level of excitement. Like chemical addiction, there was probably a euphoria at the beginning, triggered by a big win either by the gambler or someone they were with. You might also continue with your compulsion despite repeated efforts to control, reduce or stop your behaviours.

When you have exhausted your financial resources on your addiction, forgery, fraud, theft or embezzlement might become even more of an option than in chemical addiction. They are certainly on the cards if you get yourself into a "Catch-22" situation of chasing your losses, often with bigger bets or bigger risks. All gamblers chase for short periods, but the long-term chase is characteristic of gambling addiction.

Gamblers differ from other addicts in that they feel a false overconfidence or sense of power and control. You might be superstitious. You probably also differ in that you recognise your gambling as the cause of your problems.

Gambling usually begins in early adolescence for men and later in life for women.

Chronic gamblers show five or more of the following:
1. Preoccupation with gambling
2. Need to gamble with increasing amounts of money in order to achieve the desired excitement
3. Repeated unsuccessful efforts to control, cut back or stop gambling
4. Restlessness or irritability when attempting to cut down or stop gambling
5. Gambling to escape problems or relieve dysphoria
6. After losing money gambling, often return another day to get even – known as "chasing" your losses
7. Lying to family members, therapists or others to conceal the extent of involvement with gambling
8. Illegal acts such as forgery, fraud, theft or embezzlement to finance gambling
9. Jeopardising or losing a significant relationship, job or educational or career opportunity because of gambling
10. Relying on others to provide money to relieve a desperate financial situation caused by gambling
11. The gambling behaviour is not accounted for by a 'manic episode'.

As with substance-based addictions, recovery from gambling behaviour is possible through sharing with people in similar positions such as in Gamblers Anonymous, experiencing withdrawal symptoms with the support of family and friends, learning how to problem-solve and enjoying the benefits of more positive thinking.

WORKAHOLISM

Workaholism is known as the "respectable addiction" —but it incurs many of the devastating consequences of other addictions. When I first addressed my own addictions almost two decades ago, I was asked "Are you a kind person? Are you a mean person? Are you fun-loving?". I could not give any answers. I knew how I wrote and how I produced magazines. My whole identity lay in my job. I had no sense of self outside of work.

In Japan, overwork is so common, with 60- to 70-hour workweeks, that the japanese coined the term *karoshi*, which means death from overwork. Its official statistics record about 1,000 karoshi deaths a year – on top of the 10,000 people who die because of "stress/excess of work" and the 30,000 people who commit suicide mainly because they are not happy with their jobs.

According to Workaholics Anonymous, if you answer "yes" to three or more of the following questions there is a chance that you are a workaholic or on your way there.

1. Do you get more excited about your work than about family or anything else?
2. Are there times when you can charge through your work and other times when you can't get anything done?
3. Do you take work with you to bed? on weekends? on vacation?
4. Is work the activity you like to do best and talk about more than anything else?
5. Do you work more than 40 hours a week?
6. Do you turn your hobbies into money-making ventures?

7. Do you take complete responsibility for the outcome of your work efforts?
8. Have your family or friends given up expecting you on time?
9. Do you take on extra work because you are concerned that it won't otherwise get done?
10. Do you underestimate how long a project will take and then rush to complete it?
11. Do you believe that it is okay to work long hours if you love what you are doing?
12. Do you get impatient with people who have other priorities besides work?
13. Are you afraid that if you don't work hard, you will lose your job or be a failure?
14. Is the future a constant worry for you even when things are going very well?
15. Do you do things energetically and competitively including play?
16. Do you get irritated when people ask you to stop doing your work in order to do something else?
17. Have your long hours hurt your family or other relationships?
18. Do you think about your work while driving, falling asleep or when others are talking?
19. Do you work or read during meals?
20. Do you believe that more money will solve the other problems in your life?

You will be glad to know that abstinence from work is not the solution for recovery! Instead, it is a matter of learning how to balance work with the rest of your life. There are tips specifically for recovery from workaholism in Chapter 6.

SHOPAHOLISM / COMPULSIVE SPENDING

Compulsive spenders get a buzz from the process of spending, not from what is being bought. They have no respect for money, but insist that to have none would incur immense withdrawals, just as any alcoholic or drug addict would experience.

Compulsive spenders are also thrilled at the thought of not getting caught by friends, family or loved ones. Often the theft of money, credit cards or cheque books creates feelings similar to those experienced while shopping.

Shopaholics feel an intense sense of value and high self-esteem while spending, and the complete opposite of this spectrum when not.

Ken Dyer, who was managing director of a centre dedicated to treating shopaholics as well as other addicts, offers the following list of questions to determine if you are a compulsive spender.

1. Do you feel an inner warmth and strong sense of wellbeing while you are out shopping?
2. Do you really need what you are purchasing?
3. Can you afford to buy what you are buying?
4. Do you have purchases at home that are duplicated?
5. Do you have purchases at home that are not opened?
6. Do you owe money because of your spending?
7. Have you stolen, in order to spend?
8. Has your spending caused marital or family problems?
9. Have you ever been in trouble with the police as a result of your behaviour towards spending?
10. Are you regularly taking any alcohol or medication?
11. Do you eat three regular meals each day?

12. Do you find that your behaviour towards others changes, when you have no money or cannot get out to the shops?
13. Can you stop spending, without a major crisis?

Symptoms can also include lying/cheating/stealing, marital and family problems, large debts, withdrawals when not spending, loss of sleep, night sweats, loss of appetite, use of other mood-altering chemicals and behaviours, mood swings, imprisonment and even death.

Compulsive spending can also be used as a punishment, a form of debting, by people who feel they do not deserve to be financially stable.

Compulsive spenders can be treated in a similar way to other addicts. They need to stop spending, experience the withdrawals and talk about the feelings this creates, identifying why they act this way and replacing the behaviours with healthier, happier ones.

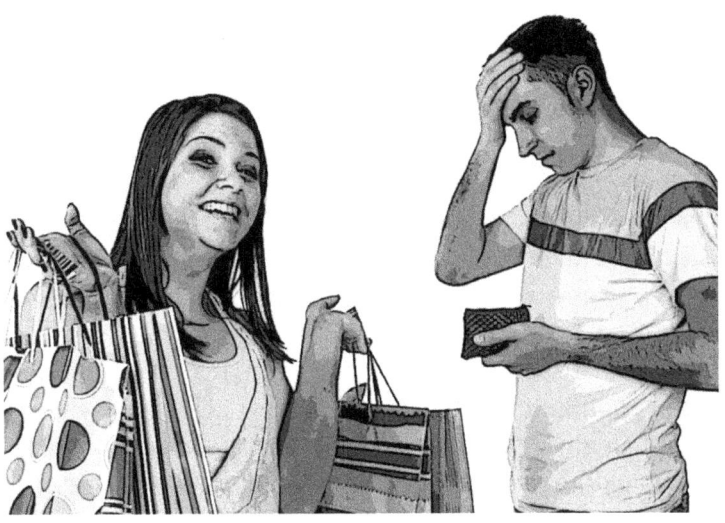

LOVE, SEX, RELATIONSHIPS

Love and sex have been described as the most powerful drugs in the world. They can, indeed, be encouraged by society – but have the same effects and consequences as all the other addictions described in this chapter.

You can be blind to the world, going through the pattern of craving, tolerance, withdrawal and relapse. Tolerance here means that you can use more and more of your addiction – perhaps more frequent sex with more partners or more violent or pornographic sex – to feel something like your initial arousal. I know one sex addict who had at least 100 partners in a year yet could no longer reach orgasm. Another put up with a violent partner "because the sex was great".

Withdrawal can include anxiety, loneliness, grief and a feeling of "I can never live without him/her". You then chase your ex-partner or search immediately for another one to fill the gap. And, of course, if you are making such a quick decision it is unlikely to be the right decision.

In love addiction, particularly, there is a feeling of "It's us against the world". The outside world is gradually cut off, as is dealing with day-to day reality. Love and sex are such powerful drugs that people held in their grip become just as blind to what's going on around them as people who are addicted to alcohol, cocaine or heroin.

It can sometimes be hard to tell love and sex addiction apart, particularly in a society which couples them together. But love addiction can involve a preoccupation with romantic dreams and fantasies – soft lights, music, knight in shining armour – whereas preoccupation with sex usually involves specific planning about the sex act itself. Of course, you can be both sex and love addicted.

The following questions to assess whether you have a problem with sex addiction come from Sex & Love Addicts Anonymous; all 40 of its questions can be found at *www.slaauk.org/40-questions-selfdiagnosis.*

1. Have you ever tried to control how much sex to have or how often you would see someone?
2. Do you find yourself unable to stop seeing a specific person even though you know that seeing this person is destructive to you?
3. Do you get "high" from sex/romance? Do you crash?
4. Have you had sex at inappropriate times, in inappropriate places or with inappropriate people?
5. Do you make promises about your sexual or romantic behaviour that you find you cannot follow?
6. Do you believe that sex and/or a relationship will make your life bearable?
7. Do you believe that someone can "fix" you?
8. Do you feel desperation or uneasiness when you are away from your lover or sexual partner?
9. Have you or do you have sex regardless of the consequences – such as being caught or STDs, Aids?
10. Do you feel that you're not "really alive" unless you are with your sexual/romantic partner?
11. Have you ever threatened your financial stability or standing in the community pursuing a sexual partner?
12. Have you ever had a serious relationship threatened or destroyed because of outside sexual activity?
13. Do you find yourself needing greater variety and energy in your sexual/romantic activities just to achieve an "acceptable" level of physical and emotional relief?
14. Are you unable to concentrate on your life because of thoughts or feelings about another person or sex?

15. Do you find yourself obsessing about a specific person or sexual act even though these thoughts bring pain, craving or discomfort?
16. Do you find the pain in your life increasing no matter what you do? Are you afraid you are unacceptable?
17. Do you feel that your life is unmanageable because of your excessive dependency needs?
18. Have you ever thought that there might be more you could do with your life if you were not so driven by sexual and romantic pursuits?

If you answer "yes" to more than one of these questions, you can seek additional literature or attend a meeting of one of the self-help groups: Sex & Love Addicts Anonymous, Sex Addicts Anonymous or Sexaholics Anonymous. Contact details for these, and for S-Anon which helps families and friends of people with such problems, are given at *www.addictiontoday.org* – click on the Self Help tab across the top of the homepage.

Abstinence is usually recommended for a year – not for life! – while you learn how to stand back and make healthy, objective choices.

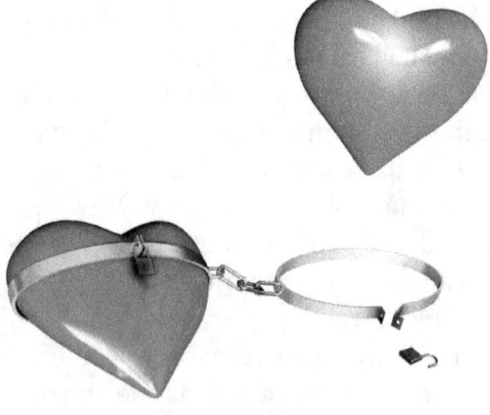

RELIGION

"I remembered waking up one morning when I was eight years old to find a catholic priest in my bed. I remembered him cuddling me and touching me at night. But my family behaved as though nothing had happened. My mother was so besotted with religion that she was blind to any imperfections in a priest. She believed his story that he had made his way to the guest bedroom after dinner."

Maria

Some people can be so preoccupied with religion and its rites that, as with other addictions, they are unaware of events going on around them. They will hear no talk which threatens their addiction.

As with work, religious addiction can be difficult to pinpoint because devotion to religion is worthy – so using it as a cover for compulsive behaviours is very effective. It is a classic case of the right words excusing the wrong actions. It is perhaps not insignificant that some family trees show a generation of religious addiction, then a generation of alcoholism, then a generation of religious addiction, the following of alcoholism and so on.

Religion can be used as a cover for compulsive order, control and a feeling of power, for forced suppression of feelings, and as an excuse to govern the words and acts of others. It can also allow the sufferer to feel safe, through justification, from the consequences of their own actions. As with all addictions, it allows the addict to avoid dealing with reality. The following indications of religious addiction I have compiled from a number of sources:

1. Do you find that, when you are faced with problems or frustrations, you tend to pray or read/recite the

Bible/Talmud/Koran instead of taking an objective look at the problem to build a constructive response?

2. Have you changed your value system when you felt it your religious duty to do so? Have you put religion before your feelings and/or your children's feelings?

3. Are you unable to doubt or question religious information and/or authority?

4. Do you see things as black or white, good or bad?

5. Do you think that God/Allah will fix you/do it all without serious work on your part?

6. Do you have a rigid adherence to rules, codes, ethics or guidelines? Do you often use the words "should" or "must"?

7. Do you readily pass judgment? Are you ready to find fault or evil?

8. Do you believe that sex is dirty and/or that physical pleasures are evil?

9. Do you compulsively overeat or excessively fast?

10. Do you put religion before science, medicine and/or education?

11. Have you alienated any family member, friend or colleague with your religious stance?

12. Have you cut back on social, family, work or other activities for your religion?

13. Do you suffer from back pains, sleeplessness, headaches, hypertension?

14. Do you manipulate religious writings to justify your actions, feel specially chosen, or claim to receive messages from God/Allah?

15. Do you get into "high" trance-like states?

If you answer "yes" to even only a few of these, you could be using religion to suppress your feelings and to avoid dealing with reality.

OBSESSIVE-COMPULSIVE DISORDER

These are obsessions (repetitive thoughts) or compulsions (repetitive behaviours) which consume over an hour a day or cause noticeable distress or impairment. At some point, you will recognise that your actions, or those of someone close to you, are excessive or unreasonable.

Obsessive-compulsive disorders are often thought of as an addiction/dependence and do appear to be similar.

But their treatment is very different from treatment for addiction, responding well to medication rather than therapy exploring possible causes. For this reason, and because they can accompany an addiction, they are detailed in Chapter 10 under the heading of Dual Disorders.

ARE YOU HAPPY?

You can use one of the check-lists in this chapter to persuade a loved one into recovery — or it may persuade you into recovery. But a colleague of mine who has a high success rate of persuading people into recovery never asks people how much they drink/drug/gamble/binge/use or how it has damaged their lives. Instead, he merely asks "Are you happy?". As they would not be talking to him unless they needed help, the question is rhetorical – but it invariably works. After all, you are reading this book yourself because you want a happier life.

If seeking to persuade someone else, ask first if they are happy, then you can move on to other questions. It cuts out a lot of the arguments.

The next chapter shows how the addictions we have just described might have started, and how identifying some of the origins can help in the recovery process.

If you have recognised yourself in any of these symptoms, you have taken the vital first step into recovery. With recognition comes the beginning of the end of addiction.

♥ ♥ ♥

3

"Causes"

Research into the "causes" of addiction is still relatively new; discoveries are being made as you read this book.

Most research starts with a general knowledge of a subject, then becomes more specific. But knowledge about addiction started with a specific form – alcoholism – then expanded to include other addictions/dependences.

Effective addiction treatment on a sizeable scale began less than a century ago: in 1935 with the Alcoholics Anonymous self-help meetings. Research linking alcoholism to genetic causes took almost four decades to emerge, in 1973. It was as recent as the 1990s, thanks to advances in brain scanning, that researchers published information on the links between inborn chemicals in the brain, how people's physiology can process them differently, and addictive substances and behaviours

While not everyone agrees on the minutiae of the research, what it important is that there is enough to prove that addiction has nothing to do with a lack of morals or willpower. It is not people's fault that they become addicted – but this book's responsibility is to show that they can recover from it.

Addiction has multiple causes and has multiple solutions – the word "cure" is not used, as the chemical imbalance lies dormant in recovery and can be triggered by even one re-use of the addiction.

Alcoholism, the earliest addiction to be studied, has been defined as a bio-psycho-social disease/disorder. "Bio" recognises the tangible, chemical link. "Psycho" indicates that it is linked with our psychology. "Social" is both because it affects our society and because some think that society helps to cause it. The "disease" word still causes controversy, although the term has helped many people to recover; the word "disorder" is more popular and perhaps more appropriate. Let's look at all the addictions under these headings.

BIOLOGICAL/GENETIC

In the 1970s, Dr Donald Goodwin and his team at the Department of Psychiatry-University of Kansas scrutinised the records of 5,000 adoption cases in Copenhagen. The sons of alcoholics tended to become alcoholics themselves; that was true even when children of alcoholics were separated from their natural parents shortly after birth and raised by foster parents. In a later test, Goodwin compared twins where one child was raised by alcoholic parents and the other was fostered/adopted. Rates of alcoholism were about the same. Environment had made no difference.

These were the first scientific papers to show a firm link between alcoholism and genetics.

Research published in 1995 also shows that there is a difference in one brain wave, the auditory P300, in children at risk of developing alcoholism in adulthood. This difference is not in everyone who develops alcoholism, and can 'normalise' in young adulthood, but it does not exist in children who are non-alcoholic.

In the 1990s, Pet scans, MRIs and other technological advances allowed scientists to look at areas of living brains light up with activity under the influence of mood-altering chemicals. In 1990 the first neuroscience – brain science – study was published showing the link between dependence on alcohol and other substances/behaviours to certain chemicals in the brain and, through them, to each other.

For example, it has been found that alcohol mimics the effects of cocaine, benzodiazepines (eg: valium) and amphetamines on the brain. This is why mixing any of the above with alcohol intensifies the effect dangerously. Alcohol also resembles opium because it can trigger bodily supplies of natural morphine-like pain-killers called endorphins.

In looking at how the addictions resemble each other at this level, we can also understand why treatments resemble each other. Even cholesterol is a complicated alcohol, which might explain some of the power of bingeing on food, and the ease of transferring addiction from one substance to another.

Understanding our brain chemistry, and the way it can 'dysfunction', also helps us to accept that it is vital to stay from that *first* drink, drug or other addiction which can set up the chemical, addictive chain.

Two areas are of particular interest. The *nucleus accumbens* is involved in the regulation of dopamine and serotonin synthesis. The *locus ceruleus* is saturated with cells involved in the manufacture and release of norepinephrine/noradrenalin.

So... imagine a substance which can boost your mood, improve your memory, reduce anxiety, banish phobias, perk up your metabolism, intensify your emotions – and help you to "just say no" to aggression, alcohol, drugs, sex, binge eating and other questionable, impulsive behaviour.

This is serotonin, a natural drug in your body – whose effects are muted, either through genetics or upbringing, in people who become addicted.

It is no wonder that people lacking serotonin's positive effects turn to anything which gives a similar impact. All we want is what people with "normal" biological systems – those which efficiently process 10mg of serotonin every day – automatically enjoy.

Imagine also a substance which can give you feelings ranging from a calm satiation to a mild high to euphoria and orgasm. This is dopamine, like serotonin a natural drug in your body which, when not processed efficiently in the brain, leaves people vulnerable to addiction.

Serotonin, dopamine, noradrenalin and endorphins are neurotransmitters, three of many natural chemicals in the body which transmit messages between nerve cells – see diagrams of the relevant brain cells, or neurons, on the facing page. The neurotransmitters affecting addiction are located in your brain's medial forebrain bundle – or, to give it its more popular name, the "pleasure pathway" – in which our *nucleus accumbens* resides.

Neurotransmitters travel only between groups of similar cells, like keys opening tiny chemical locks on the surface of each cell. There are many "locks" or receptors, each interacting with a particular substance or "key".

Between them, serotonin, dopamine and endorphins unlock to alcohol (which affects all three), cocaine and amphetamines (which zero in on dopamine), heroin, other drugs, caffeine, certain foods... The list seems to grow, with even tobacco smoke proven to react, indirectly, with dopamine. Research has also shown that even the anticipation of alcohol raises dopamine levels. This has important implications for craving and motivation behind substance-seeking behaviour, and spurs the development of anti-craving medications.

Research also indicates that repetitive actions can raise serotonin levels, reinforcing habit-forming behaviours.

Professor Carlton Erickson, neuroscientist at the University of Austin-Texas, defines addiction/dependence as a "dysregulation of the mesolimbic dopamine system" – natural 'feelgood' chemicals circulate badly inside us.

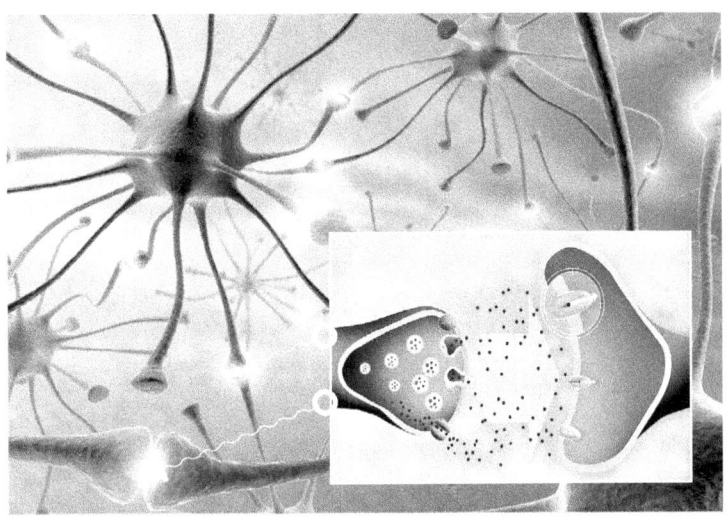

But he adds that "talking therapies" can change our brain chemistry. "If addictions are a medical disease, why do we treat them behaviourally? What is the similarity between behavioural or talk therapies and pharmacotherapies in the way they work? Simple. Behavioural therapies probably change brain chemistry!

"If this is a brain disease, and people get better in behaviourally-based therapies, then brain chemistry has to change. Recent brain-scan research is confirming this rational conclusion."

The good news is that you can raise your "feelgood" chemicals levels today, and do so healthily. Many of the suggestions for recovery in Chapters 4, 5 and 6 – healthy diet, exercise, laughing, positive thoughts, relaxation, meditation and yoga – boost your serotonin levels naturally. Positive actions and thoughts can stimulate your brain cells to produce more of the chemical.

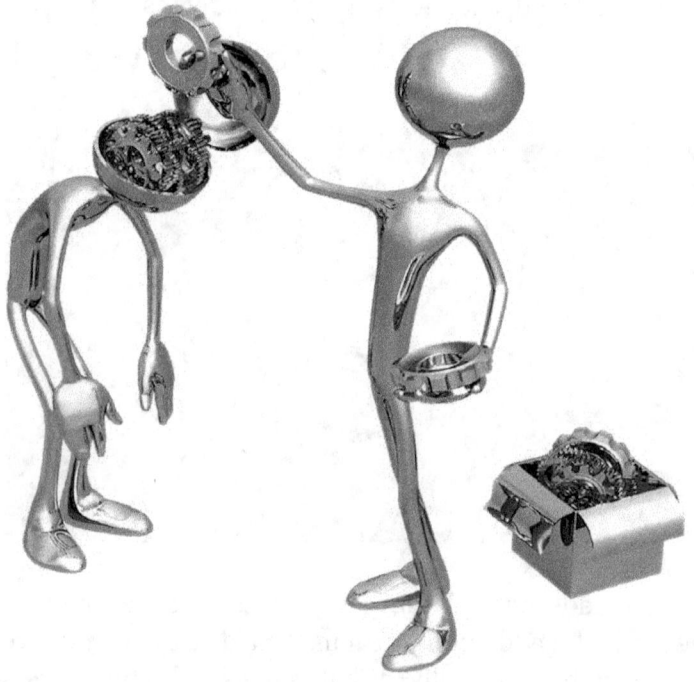

Further reading... There is an overview by Erickson at: *www.addictiontoday.org/addictiontoday/2008/09/addiction-is-a.html*. He has also written a definitive book on *Science of Addiction: From Neurobiology to Treatment*. Another helpful book is *The Chemical Carousel* by Dirk Hanson. Helpful websites when purchasing books are *www.amazon.co.uk* or *www.amazon.com*.

PSYCHOLOGY/UPBRINGING

A child with a dysregulated serotonin/dopamine/ endorphin system born into a family which provides nurture and support can do well, because life stresses rarely exceed the ability to cope. Sadly, children most in need of natural "feelgood" chemicals can be deprived of them due to the effects of abusive parenting or other trauma. For example, children of alcoholics can inherit the genetics to become addicted and are likely to have had an unhappy childhood due to the parent's drinking.

Research after research has shown that a vast percentage of addicts have had an abusive childhood. This can range from shaming messages to outright physical and sexual abuse. And the children have not been taught "boundaries" to protect themselves. The stage has been set for potential addiction and/or psychiatric illness.

I believe that all addiction is rooted in unresolved childhood grief. A parent or grandparent dies and the child is told not to grieve but to "set a good example" to his/her siblings or to "be the man/lady of the family" by not crying. "Big boys don't cry" and "Big girls don't cry" are phrases often found in addicts' childhood messages.

Children can be sexually molested, then not believed by their parents but told to stop lying; they can be molested by their parents and blackmailed into keeping quiet. They can be beaten and told not to cry as they deserve it.

Children's grief can come from having alcoholic parents or caretakers who at the least cannot show love for them and at the worst beat or molest them. It can come from self-blame for their parents' uncaring actions, from the constant "walking on eggshells" and emotional seesaw of their parents' unpredictability, and from the emotional blackmail addictive parents or caretakers can use. Children's grief comes from all types of loss: the increasingly common loss of a stable childhood, of innocence, a loved one (through death, separation or divorce), financial/academic/sibling status, dreams, friendships, familiar homes, pets, toys, of being believed, of self-esteem, of childhood itself... the loss of a sense of being loved, the loss of pleasurable emotions, the loss of an identity and of self.

Hard on the heels of unexpressed grief comes shame: "I am bad for feeling grief", "I am not good enough to be allowed to grieve", "Grief is a shameful thing". Soon, the pain and grief are remembered only unconsciously. The shame grows in the conscious. And it is a terrible feeling to have to bear.

Some people commit suicide before they are fully adult. Others have a breakdown. Others turn to addiction.

Every alcoholic I know has talked of the "high" and the mood change which came over them when they took their first drink. Gamblers enjoy a mood change when they bet, spenders when shopping, food addicts when bingeing or starving. Three types of addictive "highs" have been identified: arousal and satiation are the most common, followed by fantasy which is part of all addictions. All are escapes from their life to date.

One particular substance or behaviour unlocks each addict's individual addiction-related pleasure pathway. The mood-altering experience is unforgettable. And the addict wants more.

An arousal high can come from amphetamines, cocaine, ecstasy, the first few drinks of alcohol and from behaviours such as gambling, sex, spending and stealing. Addicts feel that they can achieve happiness, safety and fulfilment.

They must keep using their addiction, and use more of it, to get the same initial effect.

A satiation high can come from alcohol, heroin, marijuana, benzodiazepines (eg: valium) and overeating. It makes the addict feel full, complete and numbs pain and distress. This feeling is only temporary, leaving the addict with the original pain plus loss of pleasurable sensations numbed simultaneously with the pain.

Intellectually, addicts know that their substance or behaviour cannot fulfill them. But addiction is based on emotional logic, not intellectual logic. It will "solve" the immediate problem – giving a high or numbing pain/grief/fear – and addicts, not having been given problem-solving skills from their parents, know of no other way to solve the problem. This is the only route they know. This is one reason for changing your thinking, as described in Chapters 5 and 6.

Also, because addicts turn to their addiction when there is a situation or uncomfortable emotion to face, they do not learn to solve the problem by turning to other people or other processes for help. Instead of increasing their social links naturally through problem-solving as they mature, they find themselves becoming isolated.

Now a self-propagating cycle starts. The addiction is used to change shameful emotions. But being addicted and our behaviour when addicted cause more shame. The addict then seeks refuge from the pain of addiction by moving further into the addictive process. And if any adult griefs occur – such as redundancy, loss of promotion, loss of spouse – they will be suppressed in the same process, augment it and accelerate it.

Soon, all addicts need to do is think about their addiction for their mood to change. Now addicts minimise the effects of addictive behaviour – "It's not that bad" – or forgets it with "hair of the dog". They distance themselves from anyone who tries to come between them and their addiction. Their behaviour worsens. They arrange their lives and relationships around their addiction.

They start to lie about their addiction, no matter how honest they are in other areas of their lives. The food addict starts hiding food, the alcoholic to sneak in a few drinks, the gambler to open a secret bank account, the sex addict to go to prostitutes or be unfaithful. "You would drink/use if you had my problems," becomes a refrain – ignoring the fact that the problems are a consequence.

Instead of the disciplines of a "normal" life, there are the rituals or habits of addiction: knowing a mood-change will be there if they act in certain ways. Habits, instead of disciplines, become consistent and familiar. The daily gathering of "drinking companions" is a habit. A bulimic's purging is a habit. A sex addict's pornography is a habit. They need to be replaced with healthier habits.

This is a terrible time for people close to the addict. They can love the true self that the addict is. But they hate the addictive personality and actions, the words which come out of the addict's mouth. You will have deep mood swings as the addict swiftly metamorphoses from one to the other. Your hopes rise, only to be dashed even lower. You fear the unpredictability of the addictive behaviour. You lose trust. You grieve and you feel shame. You, too, need help. The would-be rescuer needs rescue.

The addict, consciously or unconsciously, picks up your shame and acts out even more often and in more dangerous ways. By this time, too, their tolerance for their addiction is lowering and they need more to get the same effect. Something has to break.

One day, suddenly, the addiction no longer produces the desired effect. Even the alcoholic can watch himself drinking as if from the outside but no longer get drunk. Or, one day, financial ruin can stare you in the face – and this time you face up to it. The person you love most in the world threatens to leave you or has left. You are in hospital weighing only four stone. You are in hospital with a sexual disease/cirrhosis of the liver/car accident

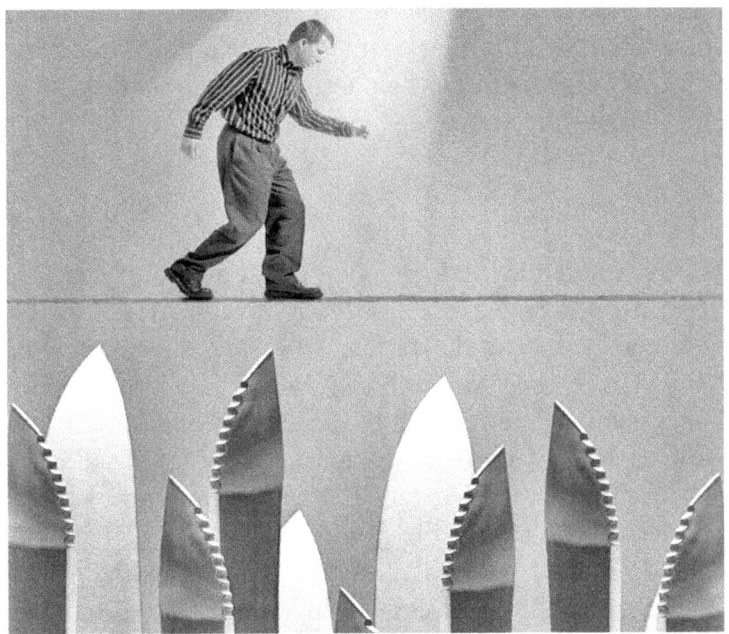

while driving under the influence of drinks or drugs or speeding to your place of addiction. You are about to be fired from your job. The social worker threatens to take your children into care... Everyone's crisis is different — and similar in that it is an emotional rock bottom.

At this stage, addicts try to do something about their addiction. In the beginning, this usually amounts to cutting back in the mistaken belief that it can be controlled, or to switching to another addiction in the mistaken belief that they can get addicted to only one thing.

But recovery from addiction springs from experience, not theory. I do not know a single addict who has not tried this stage – and anything else which comes to mind – before trying abstinence. Abstinence always seems to be a last resort. It is only after using all their efforts, willpower and intellect to stay away from addiction, and having these fail miserably, that people turn to another source for help. This is where self-help organisations, professionals and this self-help book come in.

SOCIAL

We live in an addictive society – or, to be more accurate, a society where excess is so extreme that it cannot be distinguished from addiction. We are encouraged to "drown our sorrows" or "have a drink to success" – encouraged by unprecedented availability of alcohol, pubs with 24-hour licences and supermarkets selling alcohol cheaper than bottled water. For some years now, society has witnessed across the press "ladettes" who have no shame about being drunk and risk dangerous sex.

Intensive agony-and-ecstasy 'love' affairs are promoted in our addicted society, alongside empty sex, sex as a selling tool, and the premature sexualisation of children and adolescents. School sports fields have been sold off, depriving children of a healthier option.

There is widespread poverty as the gap between the "haves" and the "have nots" widens. The education system has failed this generation so much that drug pushing can appear to be a viable career, a way of earning in the face of illiteracy and innumeracy. Often there are no good role models in either the parents nor the grandparents. And at no other time in history have mood-altering substances been so widely available, to be used as coping tools, to numb pain and emptiness and failure... until they act like a catch-22 and prevent people moving on.

Some people perceive such problems as a social and political issue rather than a medical one.

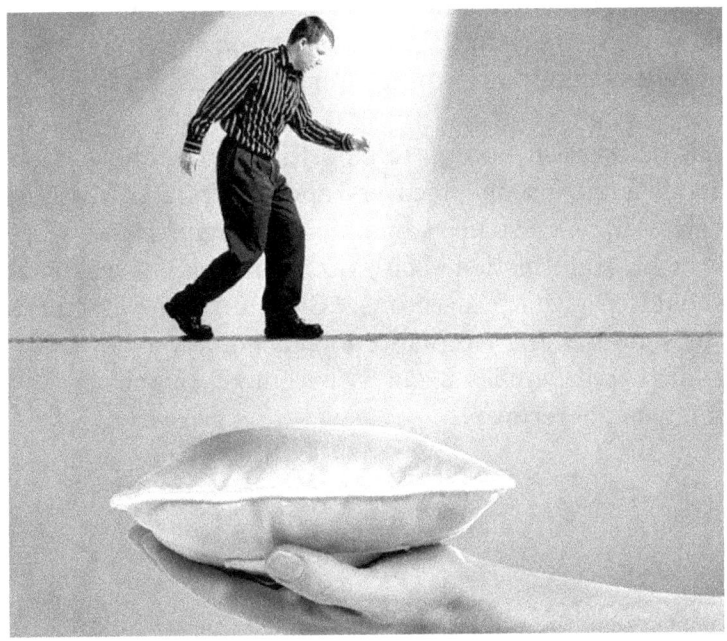

Research on the link between availability of psychoactive substances and addiction has, as far as I know, been carried out only on alcohol – but alcohol has been a good marker for the other addictions. Almost all indices of alcohol-related problems are linked with annual *per capita* consumption which in turn is linked with the availability of alcohol. This means that the higher the government's recommended drinking limits for men and women, the higher the likelihood is of more alcohol problems in society in general.

There is every reason to think that this finding also applies if drugs become more acceptable.

Surveys show drug-taking linked to poverty, particularly in inner cities. You could say that it is down to the parents' education and nurturing of their children – but who educates the parents? My 'take' on this is that addiction is no respecter of financial means – but poverty is a barrier to getting information on recovery and thus access to it.

What we need, first and foremost, is accurate information about addiction and recovery and the infrastructure to deliver it. We also need a political willingness to do what is right. Information such as in this book, for example, should be given to everyone. Change starts with three steps: awareness, acceptance then action – only then can addicts and families begin to become cushioned by the safety net of recovery.

♥ ♥ ♥

4

Self-help to a happier life I: emergency tactics

The most important thing to remember when trying to give up an addiction is that it is not enough simply to say "no". Stopping an addiction leaves a large vacuum in time and in mental preoccupation. And nature abhors a vacuum. This is when you can easily swap one addiction for another – unless you have some knowledge of how to fill the vacuum with healthy actions which will both get you through the short-term and lay a strong foundation for the future.

Addictive behaviour takes up a lot of time. For example, if you are a gambler then, as well as the actual time spent gambling, you will have spent time travelling to races, to the betting shop, to the casino, to games arcades, and taking part in social activities which involve gambling. You will have spent much time trying to get the money to gamble, trying to find money to repay losses, avoiding creditors, and making excuses to friends, family and employer (if you have one left).

If you are a shopaholic, you can pass days at a time going round the shops. If you are a sex addict, you can while away time reading pornographic magazines, inviting potential sexual partners to dinner and preparing for that, dressing up to meet them elsewhere, "cruising" for potential partners and planning your sexual activity. Time is spent both in the repetitive actions and your mind's preoccupation.

If you are an alcoholic, you will have spent time travelling to different off-licences so that you will not seem to be visiting any one too frequently, you will have gone to social events where you can drink, you will have spent whole evenings in the pub – and nights and days sleeping off the effects. You might even have served time in police cells as a result.

If you are a drug addict, you will also have wasted time sleeping off the effects of your drugs, as well as visiting different doctors trying to get multiple prescriptions, visiting different chemists for each prescription, and maybe shoplifting, mugging or burgling houses to finance your habit. Fencing those goods takes time. Meeting up with a dealer takes time.

If you are a food addict, you can also pass time at social occasions where you can eat unnoticed, or you can spend time stealing away and hiding food to eat in private. You spend hours throwing up. You might browse in health-food shops or slave over the oven, to hide overeating or starvation. You might spend much time exercising, which is part of some food addictions.

So what things would it be helpful to fill your time with? It is probably best to divide self-help into two headings: help for emergencies, detailed in this chapter, and longer-term strategies which are described in the following two chapters. Get to know the emergency tactics first so that, if at any time you feel overwhelmed with despair, rage, helplessness, pain, sadness or any other emotion – including boredom – you can get some immediate ease from them rather than from your addiction.

EMERGENCY TACTICS

In all the suggestions to follow, you are asked to concentrate on an action, by the end of which your cravings or overwhelming feelings should have reduced or even disappeared. Remember that cravings and feelings do not last, even though it may not feel that way at this very moment. They are impermanent. The trick is to occupy yourself until they go away.

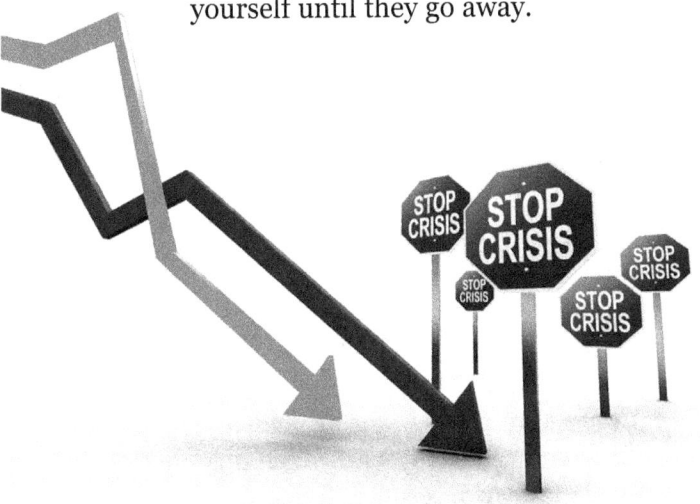

1: B R E A T H E. D E E P L Y A N D S L O W L Y

It sounds too simple to be true, but it can bring immediate results. Many people do not breathe deeply enough even though shallow breathing raises levels of the body's stress hormones, leading to constriction of blood vessels and tension in the heart. Focus your mind on your breathing so that it flows freely and deeply. This will give you some calm. Blow into a brown paper bag if necessary, or into your cupped hands if you don't have one – science proves that it works if you inhale the exhaled air.

The following methods of relaxed breathing are based on techniques by Beta Jencks.

Long breath. Keeping your shoulders still, imagine inhaling through the fingertips, up the arms and into the shoulders, then exhaling down the trunk into the abdomen and legs and out of the toes. Repeat.

Breathing through the skin. Imagine inhaling and exhaling through the skin on any part of your body. On each inhalation, allow the skin to feel refreshed and invigorated. On each exhalation, permit the skin to relax.

Abdominal breathing. Place your hands over the area around your navel and focus your attention there. Begin inhaling deeply, expanding your stomach as much as possible so that your hands rise gently. Now exhale, taking twice as long as you did to inhale, pulling your abdomen muscles in and noticing the fall of the hands. Repeat.

Imagined agent. As you breathe, imagine you are inhaling a bronchodilator agent which relaxes and widens the walls of the air paths in the bronchi and lungs, allowing the air to stream in easily. As you exhale, notice the soft collapse of these air passages. Repeat.

Waves or tides. Lie on your back. For two or three respiratory cycles, imagine that your breath is flowing with ocean waves or tides. Feel the passive flowing in and out.

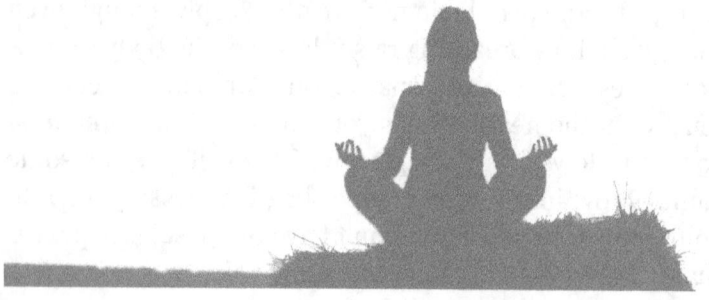

2: LET FIVE MINUTES PASS BEFORE YOU ACT

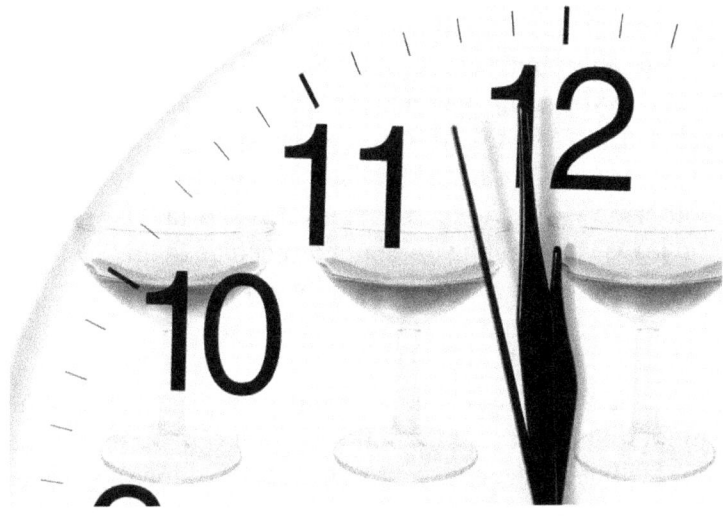

3: TELEPHONE SOMEONE YOU TRUST

This might be harder than it sounds as your 'friends' could be people who drink/drug/gamble/binge/behave addictively, and your family might not know what to do.

But it is surprising how many people whom you might have regarded as mere acquaintances turn out to be pure gold. Telephone someone you admire for getting their life together, telephone people who are recovering from any addiction, telephone the 12-Step or self-help group for your addiction, telephone your therapist if you have one, even telephone the Samaritans – you don't have to be suicidal to talk to them. The miracle is that, when you share your feelings or cravings with someone else, they usually disappear.

Remember: most people like to feel useful, and you give them the gift of feeling useful when you ask for help. If the first person you call is not in, leave a message on their answerphone, then try calling 10 more people. Even if you do not reach anyone, by the time you have finished dialling the craving will have diminished or disappeared.

Make a written note of your feelings the first few times you after you talk to someone. Did you feel better after each call? You might want to cross some people off your list. And beware if you feel grateful to someone for "bothering" with you: you don't need to talk to people who leave you feeling you're not as good as them. List the people who leave you feeling better about yourself.

3: MEET SOMEONE TO TALK TO

Meet a trustworthy friend at home or a place where you cannot indulge in your addiction. If you cannot talk about your feelings, talk about anything else. If your craving was triggered by a specific problem, try to talk honestly about it. Ask not to be left alone.

4: DO SOMETHING THAT LETS YOU FEEL GOOD

Distract yourself by playing music, having a luxurious bath, doing the washing, cleaning out your wardrobe, painting a wall, reading a gripping book. Or leave the house and go somewhere safe where you cannot relapse into your addiction – a drive in the country, a film, a museum. Preferably call a safe friend to accompany you. By the time you've finished, the craving should have gone.

5: GO TO A MEETING

If there is a 12-Step or other self-help meeting for your particular addiction, go to it. Some groups will arrange for you to be picked up if it is your first time (see Chapter 7). Some self-help groups even hold meetings on christmas day, which is otherwise a time of high relapse rates.

6: KEEP YOUR 'FEEL-GOOD' FACTORY OPEN

Remind yourself that relapsing will devastate your body's natural production of chemicals to make you feel good (see Chapter 3), that it will be replaced by a process in your body which leads to addiction and depression. Your uncomfortable feelings will last for a much shorter time than any addiction the process restarts.

7: REMIND YOURSELF OF PAST EXPERIENCES

Remind yourself of the most shaming things which happened to you while you were using. Remind yourself of how you hurt not only yourself but those you love and respect. Perhaps your employer had to fire you? Then think of how you want to regain these people's trust.

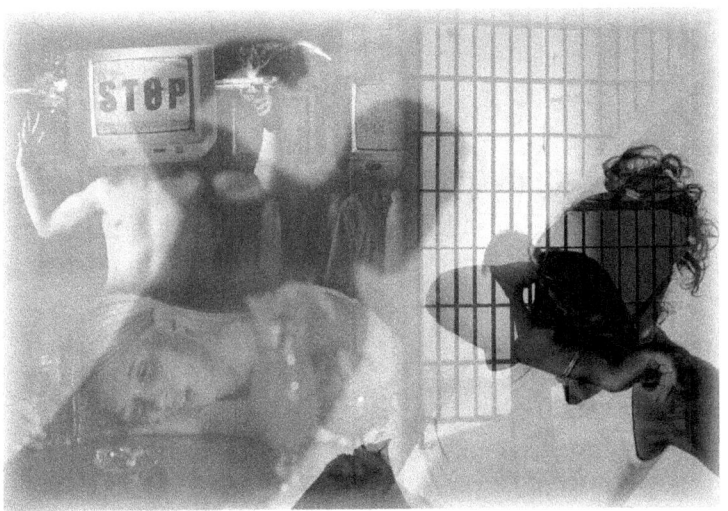

8: WRITE DOWN WORST-CASE SCENARIOS

Write down all the bad things that could and will happen if you give in. After all, why should this time be any better than past experience?

9: MEDITATE

Focus your mind on a pleasant image. Buy relaxation or 'guided-meditation' tapes to make this even easier. Buy and read a "daily meditation" book which has an uplifting thought for every day of the year. Browing through a bookshop looking for these can be a meditation in itself!

The health benefits of meditation, including lowering blood pressure, have been confirmed by over 500 scientific studies. Visualise how you would like your life to change.

10: HAVE A LAUGH

Dr Robert Holden, who once ran a laughter clinic in the UK, advises everyone to sit cross-legged in front of a mirror each morning and laugh for two minutes for no reason whatsoever! Some cancer sufferers have said that watching comedies on TV has aided their recovery also.

11: READ RECOVERY LITERATURE

Get hold of some literature, if you haven't already done so, on recovery from your addiction and read it. Listen to a recovery tape or video. If there is a dearth of recovery materials in your area, get hold of some on self-esteem, visualisation, relaxation techniques, and the like.

12: WRITE A GRATITUDE LIST

It might sound pious, but writing a gratitude list can be a very effective fix, especially when you are depressed. Just write everything for which you are grateful at this moment in time, no matter how small. Don't think, just write or type quickly for five minutes. It is guaranteed that you will feel very differently by the time you finish. What is astonishing is that, if you do this honestly, benefits will appear on paper that you never knew were in your head.

13: WRITE AN ANGER LIST

If you are raging, write an anger list. Don't think, just write down as quickly as possible everything which angers you, from dirty carpets to downright tragedy. I guarantee that this will not make you more angry — in fact, your anger will transform.

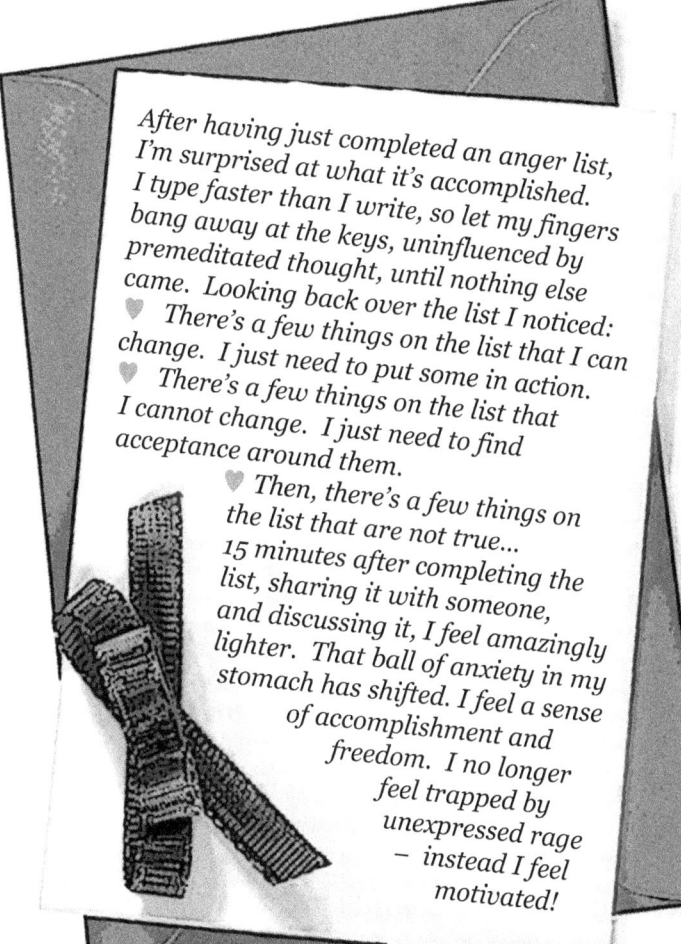

After having just completed an anger list, I'm surprised at what it's accomplished. I type faster than I write, so let my fingers bang away at the keys, uninfluenced by premeditated thought, until nothing else came. Looking back over the list I noticed:

♥ There's a few things on the list that I can change. I just need to put some in action.

♥ There's a few things on the list that I cannot change. I just need to find acceptance around them.

♥ Then, there's a few things on the list that are not true...

15 minutes after completing the list, sharing it with someone, and discussing it, I feel amazingly lighter. That ball of anxiety in my stomach has shifted. I feel a sense of accomplishment and freedom. I no longer feel trapped by unexpressed rage — instead I feel motivated!

Some of the suggestions in this chapter sound so simple that it might be easy to dismiss them – don't. They are powerful, as the letter from Suzanne on the previous page shows: it is a typical response to writing an anger list.

14: ACUPRESSURE

Ten years ago, *Addiction Today* journal printed simple steps from Leeds Drug Project on how it taught clients to use acupressure, tapping on acupuncture points, to reduce cravings. It was so successful that not only did clients teach it to friends outside treatment but *AT* staff (including myself as editor) were thanked by readers who also found them effective. These readers suggested we reprint them where possible to help others.

- Formulate a clear target for treatment – such as fighting the phrase "I'm dying for a drink"
- Rate the level of craving or emotional distress on a scale of 0 to 10
- Tap with one hand on the outside edge of the other while stating the problem as an affirmation three times – for example, "even though I'm dying for a drink/drug, I deeply and completely accept myself"
- Tap 5-10 times with two fingers on the following sequence of points, while repeating the reminder phrase "dying for a drink":
  a) just beneath the collarbone about an inch out from the central notch
  b) under the centre of one eye on the socket edge
  c) about four inches directly below the armpit
  d) collarbone again
- Rate the distress again and repeat treatment until the rating drops to 0.

Many people respond immediately to this simple application.

15: EAT

Have a snack (unless you need an eating programme), preferably one which is low in sugar.   Drink   natural fruit juices and mineral water.

16: WATCH INEXCESS   TV

Go to www.inexcess.tv on your computer and choose from a wide variety of short interviews with people who are just starting recovery, whose stories might be similar to yours, as well as people who have been in recovery for decades.

17: HALT — don't get hungry, angry, lonely or tired. These situations will make you vulnerable.

18: TRY ACUPUNCTURE

Acupuncture has been shown to reduce or cut out cravings, to ease pain, to reactivate your sluggish liver to expel toxins, and even to release your body's natural 'feel good' brain chemical, serotonin. Ensure you go to an accredited acupuncturist, preferably specialising in addiction.

EMERGENCY MEASURES: DETOXIFICATION

If you or someone close to you has been using chemicals to excess, a medical withdrawal or "detoxification" – in which your body rids itself of the toxic substances – might be necessary. This is not a treatment to keep you clean or sober: indeed, detox is akin to the ancient romans who deliberately vomited in order to keep on drinking and eating! But it will get the poisons out of your body so that you can then start on the road to recovery.

Check with a doctor before quitting your drug of dependence, as sudden change can be dangerous – it depends on how much and what you have been using. If a detox is necessary, it can be done at home under the supervision of a visiting doctor or nurse, in hospital or in a treatment centre. Medication is sometimes used.

Withdrawal reactions vary from slightly uncomfortable to painful – as in "cold turkey" – to alcoholic fits and even to death if unsupervised. Some drugs, such as alcohol, are flushed out of your system in a few days. Marijuana can take weeks. Valium can take years for symptoms such as panic attacks to disappear, as it attaches to fat lipids.

Below are some signs showing when detox is needed.

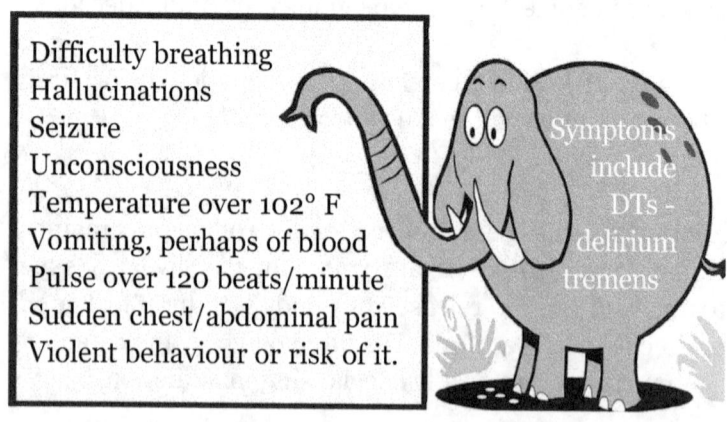

Difficulty breathing
Hallucinations
Seizure
Unconsciousness
Temperature over 102° F
Vomiting, perhaps of blood
Pulse over 120 beats/minute
Sudden chest/abdominal pain
Violent behaviour or risk of it.

Symptoms include DTs - delirium tremens

Self-help to a happier life
2: base for the future

"You can recover without self-esteem. You cannot recover without boundaries. **"**

Pia Mellody
Codependency pioneer, author, lecturer

The most important strategy for long-term emotional health – of any kind, not only away from addiction – is to learn about, and practise, "boundaries". Once your boundaries are in place, it is easier to use all the other strategies and to withstand pressures from people tempting you back to an addictive way of life. They also lead to much more rewarding and fulfilling relationships with other people.

Boundaries exist to protect me and you from hurt – be it emotional, physical or sexual. When we know what they are, they also prevent us from accidentally hurting other people in the same way, so that they can now feel safe and comfortable in our company. We gain esteem from knowing this.

So what is a boundary? Think of the boundary delineating a country. It prevents people coming and going as they please – but there are passport controls through which people can pass once their credentials have been checked. This system protects the country and its inhabitants.

If there were no boundaries around the country, it could be invaded by hostile armies.

If there were only walls around the country, such as the old Berlin Wall separating east and west Germany, no one could get in – but no one could get out, either. The fortress becomes a prison.

Most addicts are like this: having no walls so that they have no protection from damaging people or substances, or surrounding themselves with walls through which no one can communicate with them and through which they cannot communicate with others. They have not even conceived the idea of a check-in zone. Everything is one extreme or another, with no in-between.

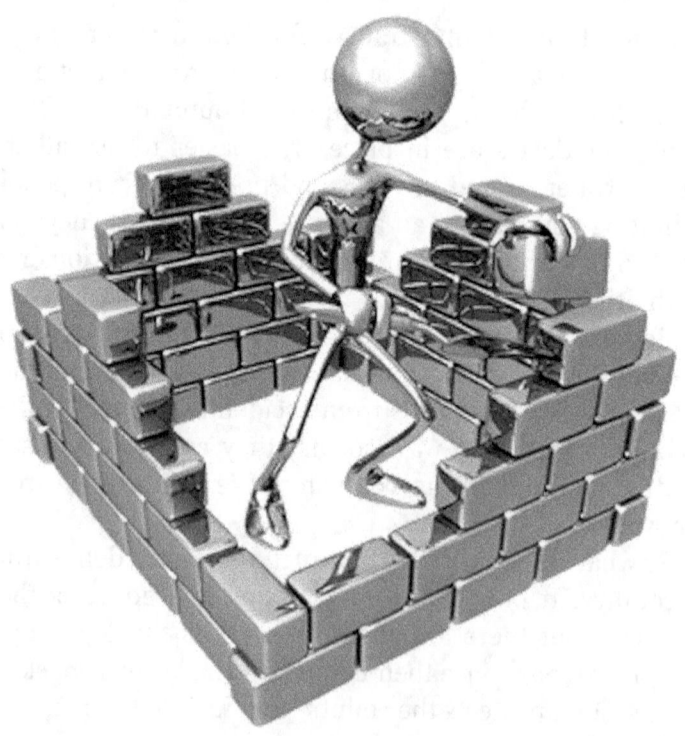

When planning to negotiate with an addict, remember that most think in extremes. You might get more success by offering options in between. Family interventionist Brad Lamm gives some tips on this in chapter 8.

The story below comes from someone who built walls around himself. Isolated with no one to talk to, he was cut off from anyone who could help him – and from those he respected and wished to be respected by.

> " *I liked to look self-sufficient, as if I needed no one. I had been taught as a child that it meant I looked successful. I did this very well.*
>
> *My wall of self-sufficiency meant that no one could see that I needed help.*
>
> *I did need help... I had no walls with my long-term partner, who hit out at me on a regular basis, sometimes with a knife, and gave me put-downs almost constantly. I drank so as not to feel this, then became so dependent on the drink numbing me that I had all the problems associated with anyone who drinks daily, including the possibility of losing my job and thus my mortgage and home.*
>
> *But I couldn't tell anyone. Ridiculous as it seems now, I feared what they might say more than the hellish reality of my situation.*
>
> *When I at last broke through the wall between me and other people and asked for help, it was such a relief! And everyone treated me with so much more kindness than I could ever have expected.*
>
> *For the first time in seven years, my situation changed. I could do more than hope.* "
>
> Sean

My own story is typical of someone without walls. Almost everything everyone said to me hurt, and threw me more and more into my addiction to escape the hurt as I knew no other way of dealing with it.

" *Before recovery, almost everything anyone said to me hurt. If they criticised me, I always believed them – even it if wasn't true, I thought I must be wrong.*

On the rare occasions I knew they were wrong, I panicked to justify myself to my 'critics'. I always tried to change myself to suit them, so that they would say nice things. In the end, most people did say nice things (except about my addiction!) but it was almost constant effort, anticipation and stress.

Worse, as I got into recovery, people told me that I was getting angry and reacting to comments that were not meant as criticisms. To me, they were. I had to learn to tell the difference.

More importantly, did it matter what others thought? This was an earth-shattering idea for me. I had never asked myself that question. Did what they say matter? This boundary question was a big turning point.

At the stage when almost everything said hurt, I attacked or defended without thinking. My tongue was quicker than my thoughts. Now I have learned – very slowly – to keep quiet, ask myself whether the comment is true (I can tell much better now) , and whether it matters; then I decide what I want to say — or not say.

I am rarely hurt. There are few arguments. Usually, I gain a lot of self-esteem. These 'boundaries' are probably the most important ones I have learned. **"**

Catherine

You can also visualise your boundaries as being like the forcefield around the *Starship Enterprise*. It can be as wide or as narrow as you like (physical boundary) and you can switch it on or off at will, instantly or gradually; I prefer this flexibility to the idea of a country's boundaries...

It can deflect anything harmful, chance meteor storm, enemy weapons or ill-wishers – yet you can beam on board anything you like (physical, emotional, perhaps sexual boundaries). You choose. If you're unsure about someone, you can beam them aboard but ask the crew to watch them...

That is what we can do with ideas, comments, criticism – anything, in fact, that enters our life nowadays, to see if it threatens our rights.

I also set other, physical boundaries about where I take my 'starship'. For example, I used to fall for violent alcoholic men who caused me so much pain that I do not wish to repeat the experiences. If I do not set course for a pub, then the odds are lowered that I will meet another such alcoholic. The pub door is a physical boundary which I will not pass. I do not even have to think about any sexual or emotional boundaries, as maintaining the physical one automatically protects these.

Not travelling through a pub/disco/casino is a physical boundary for someone trying to give up alcohol/drugs/gambling. If they do not journey through this physical boundary, they are protected from dealing with the persuasions of the drinkers/users/gamblers inside to join them (emotional boundary).

When should you use your boundaries? When you need to protect your rights as a human being and when you feel pushed or pulled back into addictive behaviour. Most addicts were never taught their rights as human beings, so some of these are listed below (from *Boundaries And Relationships: Knowing, Protecting And Enjoying The Self* by Dr Charles Whitfield).

MY RIGHTS AS A HUMAN BEING

1. I have the right to grieve over what I did not get that I needed and what I got that I did not need or want
2. I have the right to follow my own values/standards
3. I have the right to say no to anything when I feel I am not ready, it is unsafe or it violates my values
4. I have the right to dignity and respect
5. I have the right to make decisions based on my feelings, my judgment or any reason that I choose
6. I have the right to set and honour my own priorities
7. I have the right to have my needs and wants respected by others
8. I have the right to terminate conversations with people with whom I feel put down and humiliated
9. I have the right not to be responsible for others' behaviours, actions, feelings or problems
10. I have the right to make mistakes and not be perfect
11. I have the right to expect honesty from others
12. I have the right to all of my feelings
13. I have the right to be angry at someone I love
14. I have the right to be uniquely me, without feeling that I am not good enough
15. I have the right to feel scared and to say "I am afraid"
16. I have the right to change my mind at any time

17. I have the right to be happy
18. I have the right to my own personal space and time
19. I have the right to be relaxed, playful and frivolous
20. I have the right to change and grow
21. I have the right to be open to improve my communication skills so that I may be understood
22. I have the right to make friends and be comfortable around people
23. I have the right to be in a nonabusive environment
24. I have the right to be healthier than those around me
25. I have the right to take care of myself, no matter what
26. I have the right to grieve over actual or threatened losses
27. I have the right to trust others who earn my trust
28. I have the right to give and receive unconditional love.

Change your playpen and your playmates – moving to a safe environment, surrounding yourself with safe people, is an ideal boundary to keep you apart from your addiction. This physical boundary eases the others.

The "cracked record" technique usually now comes into play, as your old playmates try to persuade you – and they will try, believe me – to relapse. This technique is based on the *right* which we all have to say "no" without an excuse. If you feel that you must make an excuse, think of only one and stick to that. This will save you trying to find answers or justify yourself to invidious persuasions. It makes saying "no" to protect yourself much easier.

"
I was scared stiff of returning to my house to pick up some clothes, while I was staying with some good friends to try and sort out my addiction. My neighbour tended

to come in when she wanted (once, she appeared in my bedroom at 6am) and to throw tantrums. I didn't think I could face her, especially when I had only recently admitted to my addiction. She would use it against me.

I was shocked to be told that my front door was a boundary! That I had a right not to let anyone through it that I did not want!

"But she'll say this, she'll say that," I complained. She could manipulate any excuse I could give. I was told to reply that "I can't let you in now".

"What!" I shrieked. I'd never get away with that.

"If you must give an excuse, say 'I can't let you in now, I have things to do'. Don't say anything else. Just repeat that one sentence like a broken record: 'I can't let you in now, I have things to do'. And don't be tempted to explain what things."

I spent time at my house and my neighbour did not turn up. But, as I spent the day practising to myself "I can't let you in now, I have things to do", it left me relaxed and unworried rather than filled with foreboding. I knew that I had a tool to deal with her. It ended up being a rewarding day, and I felt good for a long time afterwards. **"**

Bryan

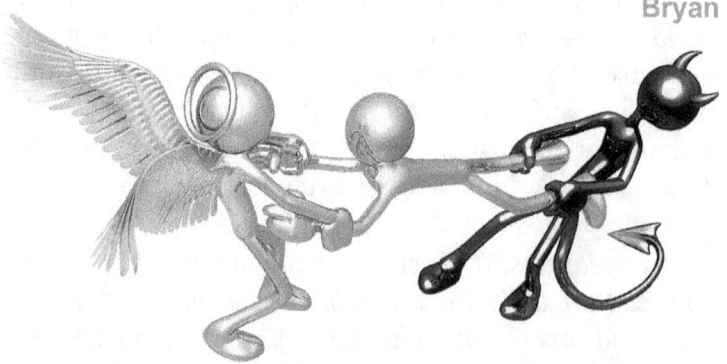

My earliest knowledge of boundaries came from addiction counsellor Sally Benjamin, in the south of England. She described a similar example of how feelings can signal the need for boundaries.

"Your neighbour keeps dropping in unannounced. You like her but are beginning to feel irritated: you wish she would call first but are afraid to tell her for fear of offending her. Then she wouldn't want to be friends with you any more; anyway, she will probably stop when the decorators are finished in her house.

"What is happening here? First, your irritation (a reaction to your instinctual knowledge that you are being invaded) is dismissed. The neighbour's feelings, which you have imagined you know, are deemed to be more important than your own. This is an invasion of the neighbour's boundaries, by the way: did she give you permission to decide what she should feel?

"The forecast for the relationship is poor, based again on what you predict your neighbour's reaction will be. You have cast her as a shallow, hypersensitive, unfeeling and selfish person *without checking* with her the basis for your judgment.

"The one thing you will have predicted accurately is what will eventually happen if you do not set your boundary and ask her to call before coming over. Your mild irritation will surely grow, creating an explosion which will probably end the friendship. The neighbour won't know what hit her, and you will feel angry with yourself and guilty for overreacting, shame for your cowardice in not speaking up earlier, and unconscious guilt for the boundary invasion to start with. This is not a recipe for self-esteem.

"Then you will apologise, without really knowing what you are apologising for. You have again not sent a boundary and are setting the scene for a re-run. You are also setting the scene for a relapse."

The feelings described in Sally's scenario are those on which people can drink/drug/eat/relapse – but are 100% avoidable if you set the boundary. It is a straightforward choice: boundary or relapse into addiction?

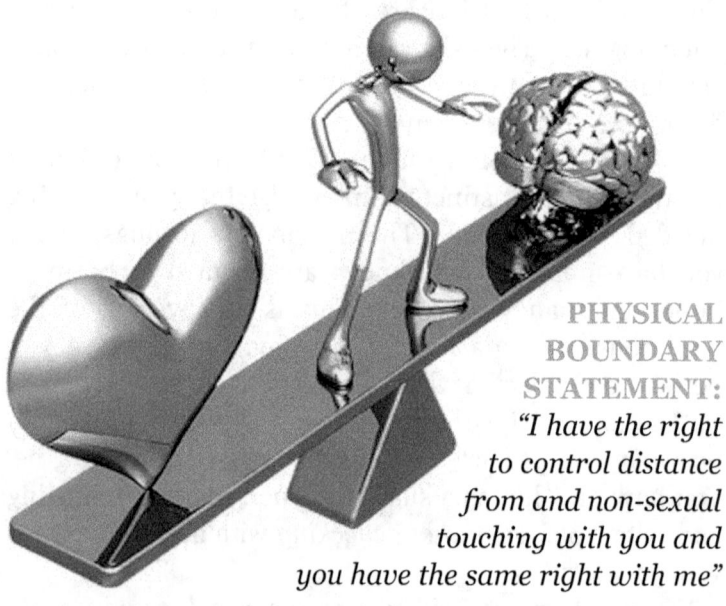

PHYSICAL BOUNDARY STATEMENT:
"I have the right to control distance from and non-sexual touching with you and you have the same right with me"

INTERNAL/EMOTIONAL BOUNDARY STATEMENT:
"I create what I think and feel and I choose to do (or not do) what I do (or do not); and you do the same"

SEXUAL BOUNDARY STATEMENT:
"I have the right to determine with whom, when, where and how I will be sexual"

Pia Mellody
From her videotape, Codependency

Some examples of boundaries are:

- ✓ "Is that accusation true?"
- ✓ "If not, what do I want to do? I'll consider if I'll respond, how, when, and to whom"
- ✓ "If true, do I care?"
- ✓ "If true, if I care, what do I want to do?"
- ✓ "I will not give my telephone number to him/her"
- ✓ "I will/will not allow him/her through my front/ sitting-room/bedroom door"
- ✓ "I will not answer calls after 11pm even from friends"
- ✓ "I will not allow my colleague to take credit for my work"
- ✓ "I will allow a hug but not a kiss"
- ✓ "I'll stay a mile away from him/her!"
- ✓ "I will not allow my sister to call me fat/stupid/mean"
- ✓ "I will not go to a pub/dealer/bookmakers"
- ✓ "Going to dinner does not mean going to bed"
- ✓ "Dancing with someone does not mean going to bed"
- ✓ "I will not drink/drug/binge/gamble or otherwise behave addictively"
- ✓ "I will not go out with addictive people"
- ✓ "I will protect my rights as a human being."

It can be useful to write down what you want to say and even to try it out on an understanding friend who will give you an objective opinion. In cases where there is a lot of fear, it might help to have a friend stay with you as you make the call or face the person involved.

Usually these situations are the result of having put up with boundary violations over too long a period of time. The build-up of anger generates fear – of what will come out of your mouth, of the other person's reaction. Do not let the fear paralyse you.

The following is a useful exercise, devised by Sally Benjamin, before you start saying "no".

A USEFUL EXERCISE before you say "no"

Having first identified that a boundary needs to be set, answer the following questions, preferably giving a sheet of paper to the answers:

- What boundary is needed –
  physical, sexual and/or emotional?
- Why do I want it?
- Could this boundary be damaging, and how -
  to myself?
  to others?
- How is it useful –
  to myself?
  to others?
- How could it be lost?
- Results of that loss –
  to myself?
  to others?
- How can it be maintained?
- Results of maintaining it –
  for myself?
  for others?

If all these questions are thoroughly answered, it will become clear whether the boundary you are considering is the correct one, and if it will serve the purpose you intend without creating too much havoc – it is possible to set boundaries on totally unrelated issues because of fear of setting the one we need to.

Remember that boundaries should be flexible. Sometimes compromises are necessary, but never at the expense of your peace of mind. And never at the expense of your recovery.

Remember, too, to keep your boundaries. To insist on a boundary one day and dismiss it the next will create an atmosphere of confusion and fear that will lead to trouble. Many addicts have childhood memories of punishment for breaking "unspoken rules" – one day, it is OK to do a certain thing, the next it is not – and, indeed, fears in adult relationships of breaking their partners' unspoken rules. Not to keep a boundary has the same effect of making people walk on eggshells around you, feeling uncomfortable about your unpredictable reactions.

It can be tempting to set boundaries in all areas of your life at once, particularly if you have had an initial success. Don't do this.

In the first place, boundary-setting is a very uncomfortable, sometimes painful, business. After all, in most cases, you are changing the patterns of a lifetime. The people with whom you are setting boundaries will not be happy with you initially (it is only initially). You will be telling them they cannot do something they have been accustomed to doing, perhaps for years.

Don't panic. They will not reject you. But, unless they are exceptional people, they will not smile at you and tell you how happy they are that you have set your boundary – particularly if it means that you are not going to support their own addictions by joining in with them.

They will argue and manipulate but eventually, if you stick to it, they will capitulate. And they will respect that boundary the next time you set it and the time after, so that it gets easier for you.

On the next pages are top tips from Jon Lavelle to help you set your boundaries with awkward people.

DEAL WITH AWKWARD PEOPLE – AND SMILE.

Frustrating situations and awkward, exasperating or manipulative people can trigger relapse. The following 'quick fixes' to sail safely through some of life's storms – particularly when setting healthy boundaries with unreasonable people – are from Jon Lavelle. There is a cornucopia of hints and tips in his book *Water Off A Duck's Back* (available at *www.blueiceconsulting.co.uk*).

Cinema surround system. Here's the first tip to try instead of the way you usually think about the person, which is probably intimidating, aggressive, annoying, sarcastic, bullying and the like... Make a picture of them in your mind which is the opposite of how you usually view them. You might imagine them as a pathetic person in a weak or feeble situation, possibly whimpering.

Before you get too far into this, change the way you are seeing this in your mind's eye.

It is likely that, until now, you have been imagining a previously negative situation in full technicolour with accompanying cinema surround sound. Imagining negative images in this way will not help you because it is like projecting the image onto a massive cinema screen which consumes your attention and leaves no room for anything more helpful.

So, instead imagine you are viewing the person or situation on a small, fuzzy, black & white TV on the other side of the room. The scene is still visible to you but in the distance. Try it now and see how small, distant, fuzzy, distorted and colourless you can make the image – and how tinny, crackly and pathetic you can make the sound.

Did you do it? Did you see it and hear it?

Don't read on until you have done this.

As you imagine the scene now, are you starting to feel different about this person already? If not, do it again and try harder, as the process should take only a few seconds when done right. Practice for a while, switching between the full-colour, surround-sound in-your-face images, then the small, black & white, crackly, tinny, distant images. You should find your negative emotions diminishing. You are turning this person's perceived 'importance' into 'impotence'. Any time you catch yourself imagining the situation in the earlier way, immediately switch to the blurred, distant, black & white image with poor audio.

If you must deal with this person again, from this point forward they will have less and less negative impact on you.

Identify verbal provocation. This is not for dealing with reasonable people, but people you cannot avoid who do not have your best interests at heart or are trying to manipulate you, other people or a situation to their own ends. Some are very clever and cunning about this; other, less sophisticated people try to twist things in a way which suits them. The first uses the precision of a surgeon's scalpel, the second a ham-fisted club hammer. Then there are the 'innocents' who do not realise how much they distort reality. There are eight common crimes:

1. using subjective slurs and meaningless labels
2. using the past to justify the present
3. using exaggerated or value-laden descriptions
4. expecting you to agree
5. direct, open criticism
6. making connections where none exist
7. using 'universal' statements, and
8. giving non-attributed opinion.

Now that you have identified verbal provocation from others, you can face it with linguistic tools such as those below from Jon Lavelle's 16 years' experience in linguistic programming.

Subjective slurs...

Provocateur: "He's such a jerk".

Response 1: "He's been acting like a jerk, has he?"

This reply does at least three things, all of them in only eight words (you can also use this response if it is you being called a jerk because you are setting a boundary):

✓ it puts the behaviour into the past (he's been acting), opening up the possibility that the person in question has now stopped doing this

✓ it directs attention to the behaviour and so away from the personal insult

✓ it questions the provocateur's evidence or opinion by turning the response into a question.

Now here's the same provocation but with a different response.

Provocateur: "He's such a jerk."

Response 2: "So he's been acting in a way that you don't like, has he?"

This reply is stronger than the first, and we can make three new observations:

✓ it completely removes the derogatory insult (does not repeat "jerk"); this weakens the provocateur's statement through "re-phrasing"

✓ it unexpectedly shifts pressure on to the speaker as it implies that they have the problem

✓ it removes 'value judgment' from the behaviour – behaving in a way the speaker does not like does not mean that it is good or bad.

... and meaningless labels.

Provocateur: "That's rubbish!"

Response 1: "What do you mean by 'rubbish' – can you be more specific?"

Response 2: "What exactly is 'rubbish' about it?"

These replies also achieve three things, as they:

✓ show that you are not prepared to accept broad-brush value judgments at face value

✓ challenge the speaker to substantiate their opinion with tangible facts and evidence

✓ force them to be specific about what they mean by "rubbish", which might then enable you to challenge their subjective judgment in a more objective manner.

Of course, you might hear what exactly constitutes "rubbish. But you've achieved your objective and clarified something tangible. If you then want to dispute facts, you could present counter-evidence grounded in reality.

And here's a third response to choose from:

Response 3: "What's not-rubbish about it?"

This reply also does at least three things:

✓ it does not argue – but implies neutrality as a minimum, and disagreement by implication

✓ dramatically redirects attention to good aspects

✓ challenges the provocateur to be balanced and reasonable; if they cannot find something good in something, it exposes their bias and calls into question their judgment in other areas.

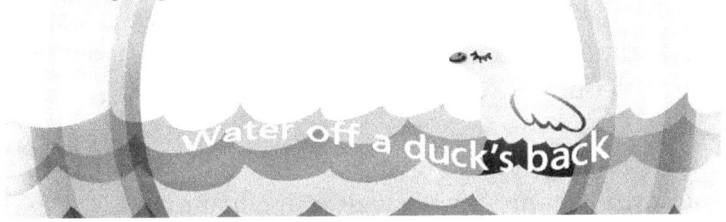

Using the past to justify the present...
Provocateur: "He's not to be trusted."
Response: "Why do you say that?"
Provocateur: "Well, he's been caught stealing."
Response: "Really, when was that?"
Provocateur: "Some time ago, before you joined."
Response: "Hang on, I've been here three years now – has he been stealing things recently?"
Provocateur: "Not that I've heard, but..."
Response: "And what exactly did he steal?"
Provocateur: "Oh, usual things, stationery."
Response: "In that case, half the company would be locked up, me included!"
Provocateur: "Right! Who hasn't taken a few pens home before now?"

Using exaggerated or value-laden descriptions...
Provocateur: "He's a bad man."
Response: "Really? You mean like Hitler, Harold Shipman or Saddam Hussein?"
Provocateur: "The personnel director's been pasted by the CEO."
Response: "What? He hit her?"

You could have used the earlier responses, challenging hyperbole. An often more effective approach is to take the exaggerated label at face value literally, and throw it back. It is important to realise that by reacting in this way you are 'just having a bit of fun'. It is best done with further exaggeration yourself and a hint of a smile, to signal that you know they are distorting the situation grossly.

Remember: you can adapt all these responses to suit your own circumstances when setting boundaries.

Direct, open criticism...

Provocateur: "You're late!"

Response: "You're right, I've been delayed by a few minutes."

Provocateur 2: "Storming out of the meeting like that was totally unacceptable."

Response: "I was frustrated by lack of progress."

In each of these situations, the responses:

✓ redirect the focus from a negative judgment to a less emotive, factual concept; you are no longer talking about monumental matters

✓ by refusing to argue, make excuses or fight back (which could make things worse), the provocateur's attack is diffused

✓ the brevity of your response signals the end of that particular interchange

✓ you are implying that you have been inconvenienced, rather than admitting that you were in any way negligent or nonprofessional.

In all cases on this page, you have refused to rise to the bait and side-stepped criticism.

THE TEN COMMANDMENTS OF RISK-TAKING

Finally, setting a boundary is a risk. The bigger the risk, the bigger the reward – but also the bigger the fear. There are 10 "commandments" of risk-taking which can give comfort and confidence if you read them before taking a risk, such as setting a boundary.

1. Thou shalt know that all growth requires risk
2. Thou shalt access all options
3. Thou shalt be willing to look foolish and feel uncomfortable
4. Thou shalt seek emotional support
5. Thou shalt be willing to pay the price
6. Thou shalt know that it is OK to change your mind
7. Thou shalt know that being rejected is not the worst worst thing that will ever happen to you!
8. Thou shalt be willing to be without answers
9. Thou shalt know that if you don't try, you will never know
10. Thou shalt acknowledge, in the very deepest part of your being, that life is precious and all too short.

Trust yourself... Listen to your heart.

Irene McMahon Cummings

♥ ♥ ♥

6

Self-help to a happier life 3: long-term plans

" A person who is master of himself can end a sorrow as easily as he can invent a pleasure. "

Oscar Wilde

Perhaps surprisingly, some of the things you can do to stay recovered from addiction can be pleasurable and fun. And even some of the more difficult actions leave you feeling better about yourself afterwards. Others might leave you with mixed feelings or with uncomfortable or painful feelings which take a while to leave – but they do leave. Working at recovery is not all blood, sweat or tears; there can be much enjoyment.

One of the most important elements of recovery are peer-support self-help groups, usually "12-Step groups". Chapter 7 is devoted to an explanation of what they are and how they work.

If you wish to consolidate the help and support you are gaining from these groups — or if you cannot get to any — there are many other positive steps which you can take to help you recover. If you have decided to see a therapist, these steps can support your new lifestyle between one session and the next. Those described in this chapter complement each other, so pick and mix as you like: try all or just a few – but the more, the better you will feel.

You will get even more out of these techniques if you accompany them with counselling. How to choose a counsellor and what to expect from them are described in Chapter 9.

Don't procrastinate — do whatever you need to do now, be it getting out of bed, telephoning a friend, going to a meeting or for a walk. You will only feel guilty if you put things off. Plan one accomplishment for the day.

One day at a time — or even one minute or one hour at a time — is all you need to think about. Do not project about the future: look after your recovery a day at a time and it will build your future. Keep everything in the day. If you can't do anything about a situation today, don't worry about it today. Similarly, if you cannot do anything about a past event, what is the point worrying about it?

Reassure yourself that, if something keeps niggling you, it can be addressed later in steps 8 and 9 of the 12 steps (see chapter 9). Enjoy what you have here and now. There is a wonderful phrase which goes "If you have one foot in the past and one foot in the future, you are in an excellent position to c--p on the present".

Start the day in the best way; be "in the moment". In early recovery, I did not have much money – but I created a safe space at home, which helped me realise that I had everything I needed *at that moment in time.* I was in temporary accommodation but I moved my bed so that the sun would wake me up in the morning. I bought the best cotton sheets I could find and realised my childhood dream of a white lace duvet cover. So my first sensations of any day were the sun on my face, the soft clean cotton, feeling my hands and feet against the cotton, knowing I was warm and dry, that I had eaten the night before... then that I had promised myself a treat that day. And I could remember the treat of yesterday.

And I had not woken up in shame, wondering if it was better that I could or could not remember what I had done the night before in the throes of addiction/dependence.

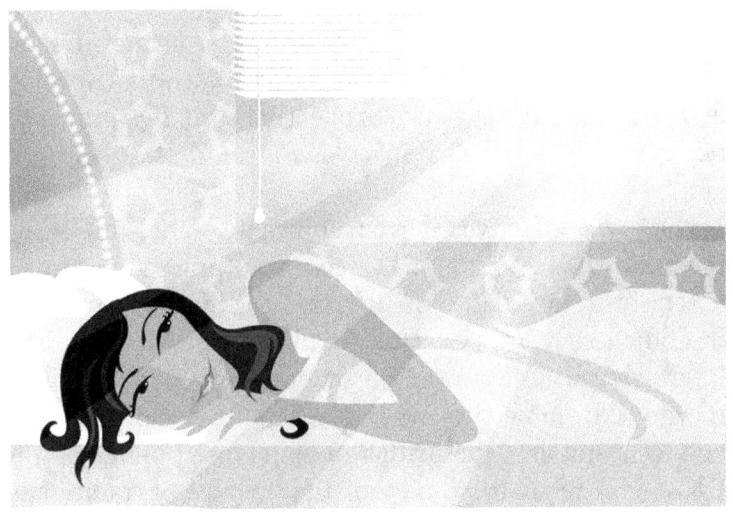

Daily treats. For me in early recovery, this was usually planning where to go to a 12-step meeting where I could feel peace, share and dispel my fears and negative emotions, meet new friends and usually go for a coffee and chat afterwards. Usually, I would plan another treat as well, but this was central. It kept my mind occupied and gave me something to look forward to. I also read those books which give you an inspirational thought for the day – but read them the night before, to dream about. All these things occupy time in a healthy way.

Don't forget to breathe properly, meditate and have a laugh, as recommended in Chapter 4. They are all excellent tools to help you to "stay in the present". Practise all of these daily, not only in emergencies. There are many books, tapes and courses on breathing and meditation, usually found under the Holistic Health, Self Help or Popular Psychology sections of bookshops, or easily googled on the web. All of these will help to ease you through difficult times.

People who want to explore meditation further, might like to visit the Buddhist Recovery Network website at *www.buddhistrecovery.org*. This also recommends books such as Kevin Griffin's *One Breath At A Time*.

One very effective – even enjoyable – help in early recovery is acupuncture. Choose your practitioner from a registered accreditation list and ask if any specialise in addiction recovery. This small number of specialists is growing as the power of acupuncture in recovery is recognised; some are now attached to doctors' clinics and to hospitals. The British Acupuncture Council is the UK's main regulatory body for the practice of traditional acupuncture by almost 3,000 acupuncturists; find one near you at *www.acupuncture.org.uk/index.php*.

Acupuncture usually takes place in a group setting so that nervous newcomers can see that the treatment does not hurt. Needles are usually inserted into the ear lobes to stimulate the liver and kidneys, which have usually suffered from having had to process addictive substances. The needles are usually left in for between 20 to 40 minutes and are, perhaps surprisingly, not painful.

As well as addressing physical damage, needles can be put in at the top of your head to allow endorphins – and serotonin – to flow. This particular aspect of acupuncture can produce a feeling of euphoria or floating when first experienced: wonderful! This also helps to reduce cravings, a physical and emotional relief for sufferers.

Because it reduces or eliminates the need for medication during detoxification, acupuncture is particularly safe for pregnant women.

Another good start to your recovery is a supplement of vitamin B from your doctor – at this stage, shop-bought vitamin B is not strong enough. This is vital in rebuilding your nervous system and is your body's natural antidepressant which alcohol and other drugs have leeched from your system.

Not only will you feel better and have less cravings but you will notice that all those bruises – which result from mood-altering chemicals eating away at your vitamin B – are starting to disappear! This improvement, too, helps to make you feel good about yourself.

At the end of this chapter, there are three tables listing natural health-care treatments, "cleansing food" to help detoxify your body in early recovery, and a "growth" diet to help keep your system balanced.

Consider hormones. Many women are blind to the impact of premenstrual, menstrual or menopausal symptoms – until they come into recovery. Newcomers to recovery often have volatile mood swings and these can be worsened at certain times of the month, when the smallest of negative feelings can be magnified. You or your therapist might be seeking psychological reasons for your negativity when it is actually due to a hormone imbalance.

Start a diary showing when menstruation occurs and dating your negative feelings. You will probably see a link. You might notice that you eat more sugary foods on a monthly cycle also. Evening primrose oil capsules are said to help even out your hormones and mood swings, as can a balanced diet (see end of this chapter).

If this does not help, and your mood swings do show a link to menstrual or menopausal symptoms, ask your doctor for a hormone indicator test. There are risks associated with hormone treatment, so you must discuss these with your doctor and balance them against the risk of relapse.

There is only one "amend" to make at this stage: stay away from your addiction. Many people, when they first stop using their addiction, feel an impulse to share inappropriate explanations or promises with their family and perhaps colleagues and friends. Don't!

If you relapse, you will have raised false hopes and they will not trust you again so easily.

In fact, most addicts will have already promised something on similar lines so often in the past that there is no reason for anyone to believe them this time. Trust is gained only over time. The longer you stay in remission from your addiction, the more people will automatically – without your trying to persuade them – trust you.

Don't make any other amends! Many people I know are still making amends years later for the so-called "amends" they made in their first flush of recovery. They shocked those close to them by revealing emotions they could not deal with, by talking about childhood abuse of which they were not aware, by disclosing past affairs, and projecting shame about deeds undertaken in active addiction. The first sentence of Step 9 (in Chapter 7) is about amends and calls first for "good judgment, a careful sense of timing, courage and prudence". Be aware that your judgment is confused at this time. But your timing and prudence can be excellent if you wait.

Don't worry about dreams in which you use your addiction, particularly if they have a bad ending. Our dreams are a way in which we explore possibilities we have consciously or unconsciously been considering. It is much safer to relapse in a dream and wake up with the awful consequences than it is to do so in real life! If you have a using dream with a bad ending, you are less likely to repeat the actions in reality.

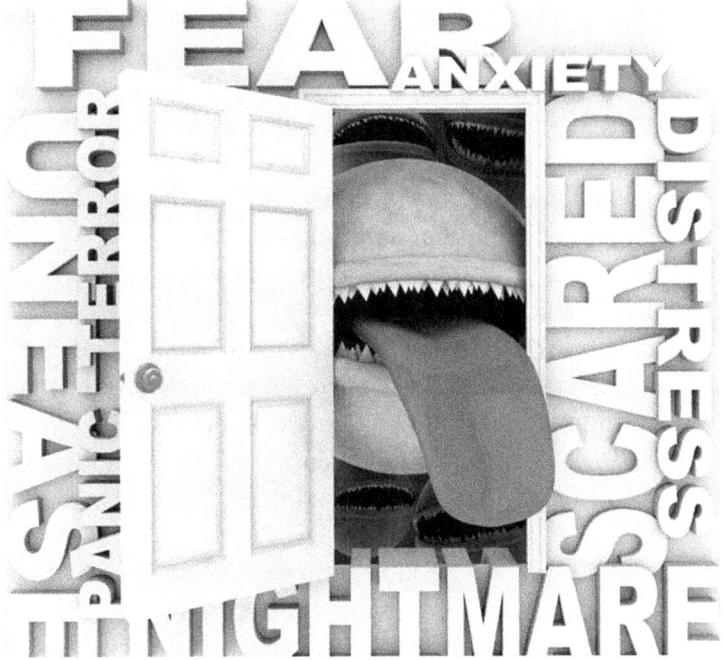

Affirmations are also good for you. Write down three positive facts about yourself on a small piece of paper and stick it on the mirror you look into every morning. Say them out loud – even though you might have been finding it hard to say anything nice about yourself before recovery. Include the sentence "I love you" as you stare at your reflection.

If you cannot think of three positive facts about yourself, ask a friend. Even if you feel that what you are writing or saying is a lie, do it. Your unconscious hears *everything* you tell it and, having no judgment, takes it in as fact. Eventually, you will consciously accept that these nice affirmations about you are true.

Add more affirmations to your list as you become aware of them.

Because you might have been insulted or put down in the first, second and third person, it helps to say and write the affirmations in the first, second and third person also. For example, someone may have affirmed that you are a kind person; say:

♥ "I, (your name), am a kind person.
♥ "You, (your name), are a kind person.
♥ "She, (your name), is a kind person; (your name) is a kind person."

Affirmations might not bring instant results – or they might, if the friends you ask surprise you nicely with their affirmations of you. But they do work. They adjust your image of yourself to a more accurate, positive picture of the new you moving away from addiction into recovery.

Now it is time for some tough work. Remember when doing some of the following exercises, that your addiction did not develop instantly and so you will not get better instantly. Be a kind taskmaster to yourself – would you ask of someone else what you are now asking of yourself?

Each week, you should feel a little better than the week before. Don't expect perfection – expect progress in the right direction. And remember that all human beings have a *right* to make mistakes.

Remember, too, that progress is slower for people who have been on cocaine or long-lasting drugs, like benzodiazepines including valium. But everyone who sticks with a recovery programme makes progress.

Take a daily inventory to see your progress more positively, and to reduce your mood swings; simply write down, just before you go to bed, the good and bad points of the day. If there are more of the latter than the former, add some of the following to the plus side:

✓ "My intentions were good"
✓ "I tried"
✓ "I was willing"
✓ "I did not drink/drug/gamble/sex/otherwise relapse".

You will always, somehow, find that the pluses outweigh the minuses. And you can usually correct some of the minuses the next day. The above list, no matter how simple it sounds, manages to balance the emotions as easily as it balances the pluses and minuses.

Don't make excuses or give a life story when saying "no" if people invite you to drink/drug/gamble/ binge or otherwise relapse into your addiction. Simply say "I'm not drinking/drugging/gambling/sexing (name your addictive behaviour) *tonight*". People are less prompted to ask you for reasons you might find embarrassing if you say it is only for "today" or "tonight" than that you have given up permanently. You have now created a boundary of *time* which – like physical boundaries – eases your use of other boundaries. (see chapter 5)

If someone continues to press you to drink/use, they have a problem themselves – healthy people are not addicted to the behaviour and prefer that you are not.

Practise the "broken record" technique from Chapter 5 before you go to any event or take any telephone call in which you think people might encourage you to relapse.

Ask for help when you need it: from members of your self-help group, from trusted friends and/or relatives, from your therapist, from other professionals.

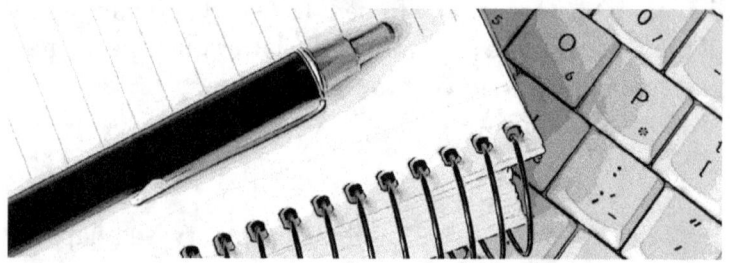

Write a goodbye letter to your addiction. Say how much it has meant to you but explain how it has destroyed your life and why you need to part in order to move on. If you write genuinely, I guarantee that this will help you to accept the loss of your addiction.

After writing the letter, you might want to read it aloud to a trusted friend or therapist, to reinforce its message and allow the feelings to come out. Remember that feelings which come out of your body are, by definition, no longer inside you to disturb you.

If in doubt about having written the letter correctly, read the comment on page 114 *after* completing it.

Change your thinking. The world will not change around you but your attitude to it can become less fearful, more confident, more trusting and generally happier. The first step is to examine your childhood messages and "reprogramme" them like obsolete computer software.

For some people, this is a calm step forward. For others, it is a freeing revelation which follows pain, anger or grief. Working through my childhood messages has probably been the single most important factor in building self-esteem and is the force behind changing maybe 95% of my previous destructive behaviours. But it does involve risk, because you cannot predict what emotions you will feel from doing this exercise.

I asked some people a few years ago to work on the meanings behind their childhood messages. Some needed to have positive and supportive people around them to talk through their reactions and come out the other side feeling stronger and freer. For others, this took a week during which their esteem plummeted temporarily. My reaction was rage, but it has built long-term esteem.

So look after yourself. Telephone one or two trusted, healthy people now and check how you are feeling. If at any stage you find yourself in distress, telephone them again. If necessary, contact a therapist for a consultation.

To start, divide a page into two columns. Fill the left-hand one with every childhood message that occurs to you, up to about two dozen. Don't analyse. Don't think. Just write as the messages arise in your memory. Give yourself 10 minutes to do this, then pause (you can always add some later). Mark the six which you feel most strongly about – it does not matter what the feeling is, just that it is a strong one. Don't read any further until you have done this.

Well done! It takes courage and honesty to write your childhood messages. It is also another step in building your recovery, by showing that you value yourself enough to do this exercise.

The left-hand column below contains childhood messages written by "Liz" when she was about two years in recovery. My interpretations are in the right-hand column.

LIZ's MESSAGES	INTERPRETATION
"Be good"	)
"Don't answer back"	) Do what I tell you,
"Don't argue with me"	) without question
"You never listen to advice	)
"Wait till your father" gets home"	) If you don't,) the threats will worsen...
"All you ever do is cry"	) ...and I'll put you down...
"At your age I had to..."	) ...or emotionally
"I never had your advantages"	) blackmail you.
"You are not like -------"	)
"Why can't you be like -----"	) You are not
"You can't have that"	) good enough...
"We are not like them, we can't keep up with them"	) ...because we are not) ...good enough.
"Don't tell -----------"	) Don't check the facts or work through your pain by talking with someone.
"Look what you're doing to us"	) All this is your fault, not ours; you're not good enough; you're ungrateful; you're responsible for our feelings and reactions.

Liz then took the most important step, which is what you should now do: she replaced the original messages with positive ones, which is what the right-hand column on your own page is for.

The reason for marking the six most memorable messages is that they usually combine to form a single, particularly strong message. This is probably the message which most influences your low opinion of yourself.

Then ask yourself "Were they right?". The answer is a resounding "no!".

The following are some examples of "reprogramming".

OLD MESSAGE	NEW MESSAGE
"Put others first"	"Everyone is equal – including me"
"Family hold back"	"I have equal rights to any other human being"
"Self praise is no praise"	"True humility is accepting myself as I am, good as well as bad"
"You're not good enough"	"I am perfect at being me" "I am perfectly me"
"I can't get this perfect"	"I can do an excellent job"
"You're bad/stupid for making mistakes"	"I have a *right* to make mistakes"
"You should have known"	"Who taught me?"

It might help to know that parents pass on *what they have experienced themselves*. They pass on the messages given to them by your grandparents, who were given them by your great-grandparents, and so on up the line. Many parents still live in the pain of their own messages, and are unaware of their damaging effect. You are breaking a long generational chain, and starting your own dynastic line!

As you start replacing negative childhood messages with *positive* accurate ones, glance at the following childhood rules and messages compiled by Dr Charles Whitfield in his bestseller *Healing The Child Within*.

In recognising some of them as familiar, you will know that you are not alone and you can start shedding them. You did not deserve these messages.

NEGATIVE RULES AND MESSAGES COMMONLY HEARD IN TROUBLED FAMILIES

Negative rules

Don't express feelings	Don't get angry
Don't get upset	Don't cry
Do as I say, not as I do	Be good, "nice", perfect
Do well in school	Don't ask questions
Don't betray the family	Always look good
Be seen and not heard!	Always be in control
No back talk	Don't contradict me

Don't discuss family with outsiders; keep family secrets
Avoid conflict (or avoid dealing with conflict)

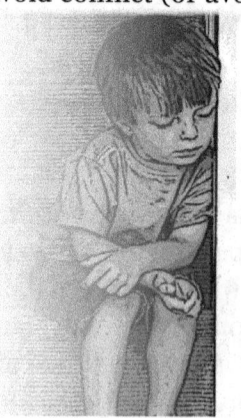

Don't think or talk; just follow directions
I'm always right, you're always wrong
Focus on the alcoholic's drinking (or troubled person's behaviour)
Drinking (or other troubled behaviour) is not the cause of our problems
Always maintain the *status quo*
Everyone in the family must "enable".

Negative messages

Shame on you

I wish I'd never had you

Be dependent

Big boys don't cry

Act like a nice girl (or lady)

You're so stupid (bad, etc)

You caused it

Of course we love you!

I'm sacrificing myself for you

We won't love you if you...

It didn't really hurt

I promise... (then breaks it)

You're so stupid

Your needs are not all right with me

You'll never accomplish anything

You'll be the death of me.

You're not good enough

Hurry up and grow up

Be a man

You don't feel that way

Don't be like that

You ----------(rude name)!

You owe it to us

How can you do this to me?

You're so selfish

You're driving me crazy!

That's not true

You make me sick!

We wanted a boy/girl

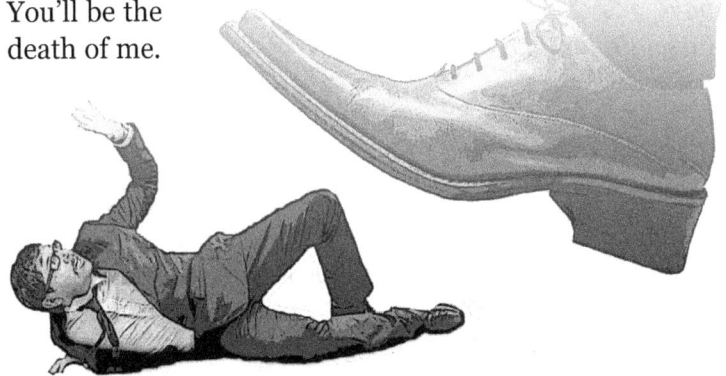

Recognise anything? The messages being stamped are as wrong now as when you were a child, and just as wrong for other children including adult children. Note that the messages are compounded by "rules" which forbid the healthy, healing expression of feelings. So we learn that we are bad, and that we are not to talk about any of it.

For some people, gaining hope of being reconnected to a healing higher power helps the recovery process enormously – perhaps because it is about something good existing. Again, that loss of hope has usually started not in the addictive behaviour but from childhood messages.

> **"**Don't do that; God will punish you." *This message, received from many people, distorted my relationship with God. He was someone to fear and avoid at all costs. Instead of seeking him for support and guidance, I tried to distance myself so God could not see my mistakes and imperfections. This played into my perfectionism: no matter how hard I tried, it was not good enough – I was unworthy. As an adult, I have turned this message around in a variety of ways: "I am a growing and developing person – it is OK to make mistakes on my journey" and "God loves me unconditionally as I am his child.* **"**
>
> *Jerry Moe*
> *Head of the Betty Ford Center Children's Programme*

Change any distorted thinking. Consolidate your work on childhood messages by questioning your current thinking – to be exact, your interpretations of the events around you. As these change, so do your mood and attitude. Unlikely as you think it, the world is a more positive place than you are used to viewing it as. There is less to fear, dread or take exception to.

An assessment of distorted thinking styles – examples are listed on the next two pages – takes several days, as you observe your thinking in a variety of stress situations. The *habit* of combating distortions can take from two weeks to several months to become automatic.

15 STYLES OF DISTORTED THINKING

The following styles of distorted thinking or "cognitive errors" come from the Center for Substance Abuse Treatment, part of the US government's Substance Abuse and Mental Health Services Administration. They are best-practice guidelines for the treatment of substance use disorders (*Treatment Improvement Protocol 34, ch4*).

Filtering: you take the negative details and magnify them while filtering out all positive aspects of a situation.

Polarised thinking: things are black or white, good or bad; you must be perfect or a failure; there is no middle.

Overgeneralisation: you come to a general conclusion based on one incident or piece of evidence; if something bad happens once, you expect it to happen again.

Mind reading: without their saying so, you know what people are feeling and why they act the way they do; you are able to divine how people are feeling toward you.

Catastrophising: you expect disaster; you notice or hear about a problem and start "what if?"s — "What if a tragedy strikes? What if it happens to me?".

Personalisation: thinking that everything people do or say is a reaction to you; you also compare yourself to others, to determine who is smarter, better looking, etc.

Control fallacies: if you feel externally controlled, you see yourself as helpless, a victim of fate; the fallacy of internal control has you responsible for the pain and happiness of everyone around you.

Fallacy of fairness: you feel resentful because you "know" what is fair but other people do not agree with you.

Blaming: you hold other people responsible for your pain, or blame yourself for every problem or reversal.

Shoulds: you have a list of ironclad rules about how you and other people should act; people who break the rules anger you and you feel guilty if you violate the rules.

Emotional reasoning: you believe that what you feel must be true – automatically; if you feel stupid and boring, then you must *be* stupid and boring.

Fallacy of change: you expect other people will change if you pressure or cajole them enough; you need to change people because your hopes for happiness seem to depend on them changing.

Global labelling: you generalise one or two qualities into a negative global judgment.

Being right: you must continually prove that your opinions and actions are correct; being wrong is unthinkable – you will go to any length to show your rightness.

Heaven's reward fallacy: you expect all your sacrifice and self-denial to pay off, as if someone was keeping score; you feel bitter when reward does not come.

The best tipoff that you are using distorted thinking is the presence of painful emotions. You feel nervous, depressed or chronically angry. You feel disgusted with yourself. You play certain worries over and over.

Ongoing conflicts with friends and family can also be a cue that you are using a distorted style. Notice what you say to yourself about the other person. Notice how you describe and justify your side of the conflict.

Your painful conclusions are based on fallacious rules. They result in misinterpretations, poor decisions, lowered self-esteem, stressful emotions – and perhaps relapse. Based in erroneous childhood messages, they never seem to be about feeling good about yourself naturally.

The following "matching" exercise is to help you notice and identify distorted thinking. Match up each sentence with a distorted style of thinking, until all 15 styles of distortions have been applied (answers at end of chapter).

MATCHING EXERCISE (DISTORTED THINKING)

1. Ever since Anna, I've never been able to trust a good-looking woman
2. People here seem smarter than I am
3. If you were more sexually open, we'd have a happier marriage
4. I worked and raised these children and get no thanks from you or them
5. You're either for me or against me
6. I could have enjoyed the dinner but the meat was underdone
7. I feel depressed... life must be pointless
8. We can't fight the system
9. It's your fault we're always overdrawn each month
10. He was a loser from the first day he showed up here
11. It isn't fair that you can drink and I can't
12. He's always smiling but I know he doesn't like me
13. I don't care what you think, I'd do it exactly the same again
14. We haven't seen each other for two days and I think the relationship is falling apart
15. You should never ask people personal questions.

Again, eliminate your distortions by replacing them with positive, accurate attitudes, just as you did with your childhood messages.

How to tell your friends, family or employer that you are in recovery differs from person to person. If people are aware that you previously had a problem, it might be a good idea to let them know that you, too, have recognised it and are doing your best to recover from it.

It is not usually wise to go into any more detail about your addiction or your recovery. Indeed, healthy people do not usually want to know complex details, only that you

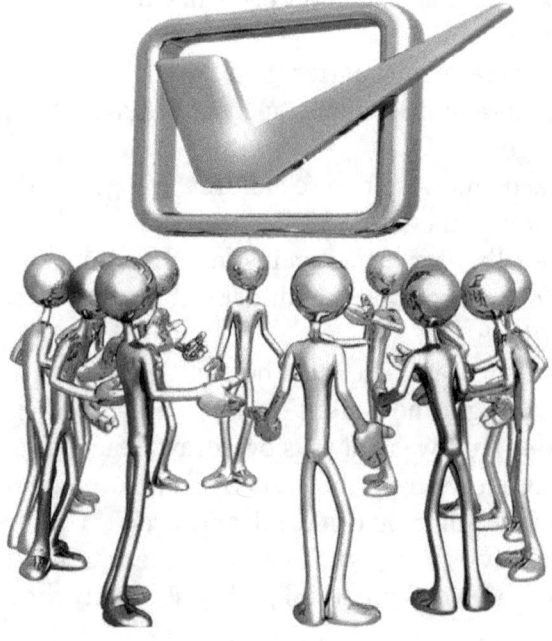

are now "on the mend". I remember trying to tell a past employer that I had just started recovery. He stopped me almost mid-sentence and said "All I care about is that you feel happier now".

Another old friend, Laurence, with whom I had lost touch during the worst of my addictive behaviour and whom I also contacted in early recovery, simply said "But I always loved you; I was just concerned about you hurting yourself with your behaviour". Hopefully, you will have similar unexpected caring experiences.

If people do want to know more, be honest with them. This applies particularly to your family – this is probably make-or-break time for your family relationships.

If you have children, you need to let them know that you have changed. No matter how young they are, they have been affected by your addictive behaviour. It might be an idea to wait until you have been a little while in recovery, by which time they will have noticed a change and can believe what you tell them. Also, if you had relapsed after telling them too soon, you would have raised false hopes and broken their trust. They will find it harder to believe you in the future.

Before you talk to your children, read Chapter 9 which is about trying to prevent children from following in their parents' addictive footsteps. Apply its principles to your own children. Remember the false childhood messages and faulty thinking in this chapter, and try never to pass them on to your children. Give them the positive replacement messages instead. Mature together.

And remember that children do as their parents do, rather than what they say. Your own healthy recovery is the best preparation for life for both of you.

Encourage your partner to attend Al-Anon, Alateen, Families Anonymous, Gam-Anon or other organisations which help the families of addictive people. If they do not like the meetings, they can at least pick up some literature to give them an understanding of what is happening and how they can be supported throughout your recovery.

Choose your career carefully. It is important to most people to have a career rather than "a job", but it is even more important to people in recovery. It has been said that up to 80% of all grief comes from being in the wrong job. The difference between a career and a job is that the first offers hope and fulfilment, the second offers only money. You will lose that money if you relapse on the unhappiness the job brings.

Having said that, many people in the first year or two of recovery take on simple work, usually volunteer work. This is ideal as it allows you to cope with all your new learning and life skills, practise managing your mood swings, and process the new emotions you are feeling. It allows you to practise bonding healthily with other people, perhaps for the first time. It means that you can concentrate on you and your needs and start to get a sense of self from what is within you, independent of the job you hold. This is particularly important for people with workaholic tendencies.

If you are in a high-stress job and cannot or do not wish to leave it, delegate or cut back on some of your responsibilities. Plan how much work you can achieve in office hours and stick to it. Because your mind is now clearer, you might find that some work is unnecessary, and that you take less time to achieve more of the necessary work.

Finally, choose the job sector you enter carefully. Working in a drinks-related industry, for example, is not a good idea; publicans and bar staff have the highest death rates from alcohol-related problems. Close behind are doctors, seafarers and lawyers. If you happen to be a qualified doctor or lawyer, there are special self-help groups for you (see Chapter 7).

Don't rush into a relationship. Try to wait for a year – the healthier you are in your recovery, the healthier a partner you will choose. In early recovery, it is likely you will only repeat past experiences. Or that you will fall for a "13 Stepper", an oldtimer in self-help programmes who is adept at seducing vulnerable newcomers. S/he usually does not relapse on this – their victims often have.

Also, in early recovery it is easy to transfer your addiction from whatever it has been to sexual activity or a specific person. You can find yourself spending time on them that you should be spending on your recovery.

You can block out feelings you need to experience by instead feeling a high from "love", lust and the dream of romance. You have merely swapped one addiction for another.

Addiction freezes personality development so that, no matter what your chronological age is, you are probably the emotional age of when you first starting using your addiction – usually this is the emotional age of an adolescent. For example, you might find yourself blushing and feeling awkward like you did when a teenager.

You should be spending the first year of recovery maturing and advancing your interpersonal skills before you try to build a serious relationship.

If you were already in a relationship before recovery, it is advised that you don't rush out of it! Again, unless you work through your issues, you could be doomed to repeat your unhappy patterns. The exception is that you must escape from abusive partners.

On the next page is a questionnaire – compiled by Wayne Kritsberg of *Family Integration Systems* – to help you to determine if you have become involved in a codependent, addictive, relapse-prone relationship.

ARE YOU IN A CODEPENDENT RELATIONSHIP?

1. Do you place your partner's needs ahead of yours?
2. Have you ever hit or been hit by your partner?
3. Are you afraid to tell your partner when your feelings are hurt?
4. Does your partner tell you how to dress?
5. Do you smile when you are angry?
6. Do you have difficulty establishing personal boundaries and keeping them?
7. Is it difficult to express your true feelings to your partner?
8. Do you feel nervous and uncomfortable when alone?
9. Do you feel rejected when your partner is spending time with friends?
10. Do you feel shame when your partner makes a mistake?
11. Do you have sex when you do not want to?
12. Do you withhold sex to get even with your partner?
13. Do you think your partner's opinion is more important than your own?
14. Do you rely on your partner to make most of the decisions in the relationship?
15. Do you become very upset when your partner does not follow your plan?
16. Are you afraid to let your partner really know what you are feeling?
17. Do you keep silent to keep the peace?
18. Do you feel you give and give and get little or nothing in return?
19. Do you freeze up when in conflict with your partner?
20. Are you unhappy with your friendships?
21. Do you often find yourself saying "It's not that bad"?

22. *Do you feel you are "stuck" in this relationship?*
23. *Must you control your emotions most of the time?*
24. *Do you lose control of your emotions during conflict?*
25. *Do you feel that your relationship would fall apart without your constant efforts?*

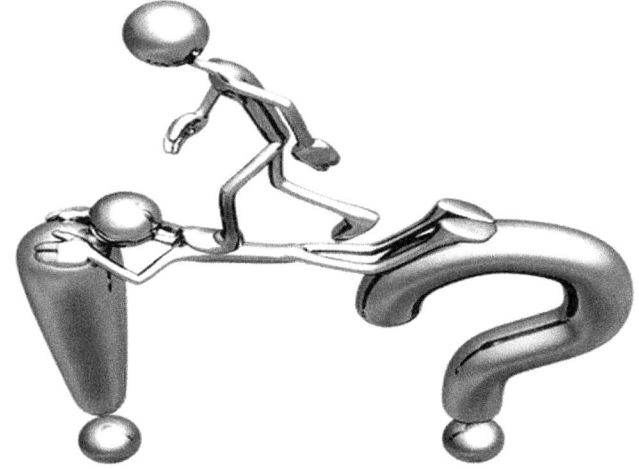

A score of five or more "yes" answers indicates that you might be or have been in a codependent relationship. The more "yes" answers, the more dysfunctional the relationship.

As mentioned, if you are already in a relationship, it is usually advised not to make any decisions about it until a year of recovery has passed. There are exceptions, such as being in a violent relationship or with a partner tempting you to relapse. Women tend to relapse in response to a using male partner's encouragement more than men relapse in response to a female partner.

Getting into, or out of, a relationship can be pivotal in most people's lives. Give it the importance it deserves by discussing it thoroughly with people you trust before taking any action.

Christmas and New Year are highly stressful events
for anyone, as the high suicide rates at this time of year
show. With recovering people, the stress is reflected in the
high rates of relapse in late December and early January,
and relapses in late January from complacency at having
got through the first period.

Stress comes from having high expectations of Christmas
and New Year, then having them disappointed. It comes
from memories of shameful addictive behaviour during
past Christmases and New Years. It comes from images
all over the media of ideal happy families, something
which addicts have usually either lost or never had in the
first place. An aching emptiness opens – but you need not
fill it with addictive substances or behaviours.

Addicts can also feel that they must present a perfect
image at this time, and this can be an unnatural strain.

One treatment centre says that its clients who are
mothers carry overwhelming guilt as they see history
repeat itself. Many of them overcompensate by shoplifting
expensive clothes and toys – which confuses the children.

So what preparations can you make to guard against
relapse – and perhaps even have a good time?

♥ Meet with some friends as early as November and
discuss your fears. Share your fears at self-help meetings
and with your therapist, if you have one.

♥ Plan the event(s) well ahead. Account for as much
as possible of your time with positive activities. Where do
you want to spend Christmas? Do you want to spend it
alone? With friends, family or other single members of
your fellowship? Ask them, then enjoy planning together.

♥ Keep things low key.

♥ If necessary, use emergency tactics in Chapter 4.

♥ Some self-help groups hold meetings on the eve

and day of Christmas and New Year. Go if one is available. Some groups also hold a New Year's eve dance.

♥ If going away, take recovery literature and tapes with you. Take soft drinks also. Serve your own drinks so no one can "spike" them. If things get too much, go for a walk or to a room with privacy. Have a plan of escape ready in case things get worse.

♥ If you must go to events of which you are fearful, ensure you have the means to get away quickly. Ask a friend to collect you at a certain hour. Have money for a telephone call to ring them sooner if necessary. Have the money for a cab. Have a good excuse prepared. If you trust the host or a fellow guest, let them know that you must put your recovery first.

♥ Stock up with lots of exotic soft drinks, so there is no excuse to go to an off-licence or public bar. Garnish them so they look special.

By surviving one Christmas and New Year, you learn that you can enjoy yourself without your addiction. You have set up a new "building block" for future years. And I guarantee that the following year will be easier, because you will have good memories and experience to draw on.

There are more hints and tips on getting through this perilous time of year at *www.addictiontoday.org/ addictiontoday/2008/10/help-clients-to-survive-the-festive-season.html*

Other holidays can be made easier if you find out in advance where nearby self-help meetings are held, so you can express fears and spend time with "locals" in recovery. This is a huge advantage which members of self-help groups have that the general public does not: a way to meet local people quickly, with friendship and lots in common. You can also organise your entire holiday with an agency specialising in vacations for people in recovery. If you would like to holiday abroad, knowing that you are not risking your sobriety, try these websites:

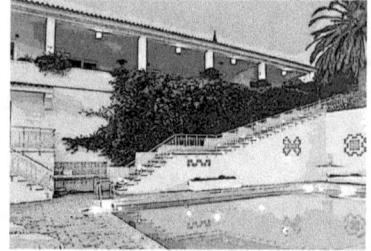

www.soberholidays.net

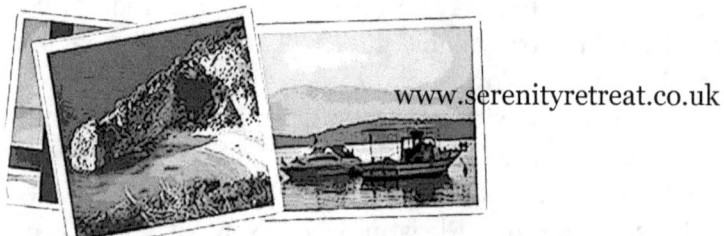

www.serenityretreat.co.uk

www.sobercelebrations.com

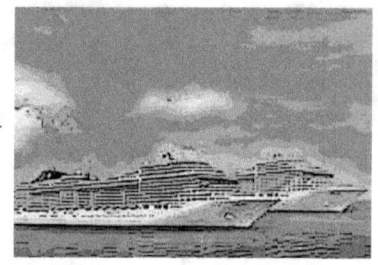

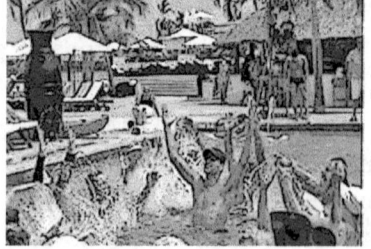

www.sobervacations.com

Also:
www.sobertravelers.org

Help your body to recover. Some of the main biochemical imbalances experienced by people with addictive disorders are listed below by Dr Mark Atkinson.

Neurotransmitter imbalances, including those of serotonin, dopamine and acetylcholine. Address these using specific amino acid supplements, nutrient therapy and the judicious use of prescribed medication; this can be enhanced even further with acupuncture.

Dysglycemia – fluctuating blood-sugar levels – is a very common contributor to mood swings, depression, irritability and poor concentration. This can be addressed by eating a nutrient-dense whole-foods diet high in vegetables, whole grains, fruits, nuts and seeds and high-quality protein, and low in processed foods, transfatty acids, sugar and caffeine. The mineral chromium is also useful to stabilise blood sugar.

Mineral/vitamin/essential-fatty acid imbalances: nutrient deficiencies are very common in people with substance addictions. These can be addressed using nutritional supplements and a tailored diet.

Food intolerances/sensitivities are particularly common in alcoholics: wheat, dairy and sugar are the most common. Remove the triggering foods for a time while underlying issues, such as leaky gut syndrome, are addressed.

Adrenal fatigue: many patients with addictive illness are exhausted and find themselves more able to do the necessary psychological work of recovery once receiving treatment for adrenal fatigue. Hypothyroidism can sometimes co-exist with this, so should be checked for.

You can read Dr Atkinson's holistic approach to recovery from addictive disorders at: *www.addictiontoday.org/ addictiontoday/2010/04/integrated-holistic-approach-to-addictive-disorders.html.*

Help your body to recover. The following three lists of natural healthcare treatments – starting with "cleansing" foods for your body in early recovery then a "growth" diet to keep your system balanced – were devised by John Tindall MCSP, SRP, MRCHM, a London-based chinese-medicine specialist in substance abuse and HIV. You can read more about his work or make an appointment here: *www.yuantmc.co.uk/clinic/clinicmenu.htm.*

Detoxification period: cleansing food:

1. Fresh fruit and vegetables – cleansing
2. Wholegrains, eggs, fish more than meat and milk which burden the liver and kidneys
3. No greasy and fried foods which harm liver, skin and circulation
4. No sugar or refined flour products as they leech vitamins and minerals
5. Plenty of water and herbal tea
6. No tea or coffee, which leech vitamins and minerals.

Growth diet:

1. Protein and carbohydrate separate
2. 80% alkaline foods
3. No fluid with meals
4. 75% of meal should be water
5. Chew well
6. No emotional "pigging out"; eat only when hungry
7. Eat regularly.

Natural health-care treatments:

Acupuncture	Especially for acute withdrawal symptoms and chronic problems post-detoxification
Shiatsu	Body work to release blockages and invigorate Qi energy & blood circulation
Relfexology	Foot massage especially useful for insomnia, headaches, withdrawal pains and digestive disorders
Hydrotherapy	Hot and cold baths for leg and back pains and to reduce acidosis
Essential oils	Very good for relaxation and muscle aches and pains. The most commonly used are lavender, ylang ylang and rosemary – use four drops of each in your bath
Herbal teas	To cleanse and restore the internal chemistry of the body
Detox tea	Camomile 1 part, scullcap 1, peppermint 1, catmint 1, yarrow 1, elder 1, vervain 1 Dose: 1tsp of boiling water x 3 daily
Sleep tea	Camomile 1 part, motherwort 1, scullcap 1, passiflora 1, damiana 1, red clover 1, hop 0.25, lime flowers 1. Dose: 1 tsp of mixture/cup of boiling water x 2 in evening
Moxibustion	For cold, weak, tired symptoms in chronic abusers. Is an ancient chinese practice of warming points of the body to improve circulation, reduce pain and energise the internal systems
Western exercise	To promote lymphatic & blood circulation and stimulate the release of endorphins. Fostering communication, team spirit and discipline. Examples: circuit training, skipping, running, volley/basket ball, etc

Eastern exercise	*Qi Gong* to integrate the mind, body and breathing in simple meditative movements or postures, to reach the highest level of realisation *Yoga* to release physical & mental tension, to attain a raised consciousness.
Vitamins, minerals:	To address the deficiency created by consistent drug abuse.
Vitamin C	2g daily for adrenal and liver function, antibody formation, counter-acidosis and infections and capillary blockage
Vit B Complex	Nervous tissue, liver and skin
Vitamin E	400iu daily prevents destruction of vital fats, produces fatty hormones, improves liver function, reduces scars (if high blood pressure, do not exceed 50iu daily)
Vitamin A	10,000iu daily improves eliminative function of the skin & mucus membranes, improves liver function, tones itchy skin
Vitamin D	1,000iu daily improves absorption of calcium and thus aids healing of nerves, bones and muscle
Zinc	30mg daily improves reaction to stress, inflammation, low fertility
Iron	10mg for anaemia (yellow dock)
Manganese	Improves use of vitamin F sterility, hyperactivity, bone and joint changes and pituitary weakness
Calcium & magnesium	For bone pains, nerves. Dolomite 300mg daily
Relaxation	Autogenics relaxing exercise, meditation including transcendental meditation, biofeedback.

See a doctor to check your health. Reality usually turns out to be much better than your fears. Also, many illnesses resulting from addiction are curable – even the liver can repair itself, unless it is at end-stage cirrhosis. You deserve to have your body looked after. Addiction is about avoiding reality, so facing up to this reality gives the addiction less of an excuse to come back.

If you do have a serious b r a i n or liver problem, there is a recent m e d i c a l treatment which could be worth checking out:

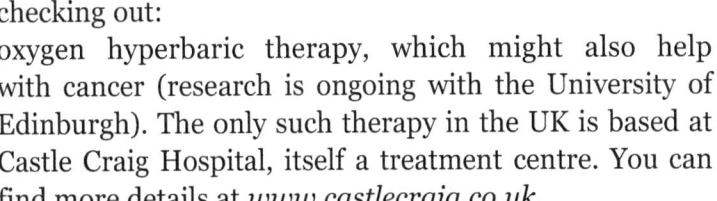

oxygen hyperbaric therapy, which might also help with cancer (research is ongoing with the University of Edinburgh). The only such therapy in the UK is based at Castle Craig Hospital, itself a treatment centre. You can find more details at *www.castlecraig.co.uk*.

If your own doctor does not understand about addiction, ask an organisation such as the Medical Council on Alcoholism in the UK (*www.m-c-a.org.uk*) or the American Society of Addiction Medicine in the US (*www. asam.org*) for a doctor in your area who understands about, and is sympathetic to, recovery from addiction.

The Addiction Recovery Foundation plans to make a list available (updates at *www.addictiontoday.org*).

Finally, when for some reason none of the techniques in this or the previous chapters seem to be enough – go to a self-help meeting or seek professional help. The details are in the next chapters.

Seeking professional help is not a 'failure' on your part but, rather, a courageous and intelligent acknowledgment that you have an illness which requires indepth care.

♥ ♥ ♥

Solutions:

Goodbye letter (see page 92) — you know that you have written this genuinely if it reads like a goodbye letter to a lover.

Distorted thinking (see page 101) —

1. Overgeneralisation
2. Personalisation
3. Fallacy of change
4. Heaven's reward fallacy
5. Polarised thinking
6. Filtering
7. Emotional reasoning
8. Control fallacies
9. Blaming
10. global labelling
11. Fallacy of fairness
12. Mind reading
13. Being right
14. Catastrophising
15. Shoulds.

12 Step recovery: first, largest, worldwide

Some time ago, the presenter on a US television chat show asked diplomat Henry Kissinger – then at the height of his fame and power – what was the most valuable export the US had given to the world. "Alcoholics Anonymous," came his reply.

When I wrote the first edition of this book, UK researchers and policymakers were reluctant to accept the efficacy of 12-Step programmes and therapeutic treatment which linked skills to it – despite millions of people having reclaimed their lives with its support, and despite its popularity in the US. The situation has since improved, with Alcoholics Anonymous and other 12-Step programmes recommended in government policies (see chapter 9).

Twelve-Step programmes, Alcoholics Anonymous, Narcotics Anonymous, Cocaine Anonymous and recovery are terms which have recently been popularised. Much of this is due to celebrities hitting the media headlines with their addiction – and recovery. Characters in TV programmes and films drop the words casually. Early mentions came in the 1980s TV detective show *Cagney & Lacey*, where a lead character regularly went to AA meetings. In 1992, Tim Robbins' character in *The Player* announced casually that he was dropping into an AA meeting not because he had an alcohol problem but to meet film-industry contacts there. In the 2007 romance *My Name Is Sarah*, a nonalcoholic woman accidentally attends AA meetings.

Other films featuring aspects of addiction and the 12 Steps include:

ⓘ *The Lost Weekend* 1945 – perhaps the best-known film about alcoholism; Ray Milland plays a writer who goes on a binge and ends up in Bellevue hospital/asylum

ⓘ *My Name is Bill W* 1989 – about the founders of AA

ⓘ *Opening Night* 1977 – how alcoholics surround themselves with enablers who help them to drink

ⓘ *28 Days* 2000 – Sandra Bullock gets clean and sober in rehab, learns the 12 Steps and starts a new life

ⓘ *Clean and Sober* 1988 – Michael Keaton cons his way into rehab, realises he is an addict, recovers with new friends

ⓘ *Clean* 2004 – heroin overdose, dead using-companions, losing custody of son, methadone addiction... then recovery

ⓘ *Skin Deep* 1989 – writer moans, suffers, is impotent, can't write, considers suicide... until shrink says: Stop drinking

ⓘ *Under the Volcano* 1984 – within every drunk is a person with self-respect trying to get free

ⓘ *The Basketball Diaries* 1995 – drug addiction in school

ⓘ *The Boost* 1988 – portrait of cocaine addiction

ⓘ *Only When I Laugh* 1981 – alcoholic actress struggles to quit the bottle, and her relationship with her daughter

ⓘ *The Verdict* 1982 – lawyer whose lost job, divorce and disbarment hearing are all traceable to his alcoholism

ⓘ *Days of Wine and Roses* 1962 – husband and wife drink alcoholically, he gets sober, she cannot, implications

ⓘ *Leaving Las Vegas* 1996 – dying from alcoholism

ⓘ *A Long Day's Journey Into Night* 1962 – a dope-addicted wife whose alcoholic son would rather destroy all around him than show the deep affections he feels.

There are now 12-Step programmes for almost every addiction. But what are they and how can they help people to recover?

All 12-Step programmes are based on the earliest one, Alcoholics Anonymous, which was founded in 1935 by stockbroker Bill Wilson and surgeon Robert – "Dr Bob" – Smith. Both had tried unsuccessfully for years to give up their addiction to alcohol – and succeeded only when they accidentally met and talked to each other about it.

This is why addiction is often called "the only disease which can be cured by talking".

Bill Wilson and Dr Bob decided to spread the message about what had worked for them, in the hope of helping other people with similar addiction problems. The infant society set down its experience in a book which reached the public four years later. At this time, the recoveries numbered about 100 people.

The book was simply called *Alcoholics Anonymous*, often referred to as "The Big Book", and from it the fellowship took its name. Its basic text remains unchanged through three editions, many reprints and millions of sales. It gives a history of AA and a clear understanding of alcoholism, with a way out of addiction. Personal stories were added after the second edition, differing enough for any reader with a severe drinking problem to identify with at least one of them. The book spurred alcoholics to flock to AA in their tens of thousands. There are now millions of people in AA worldwide.

When AA's founders were 15 years sober, they collated the experience and knowledge gained from their own sobriety and from other members in the quickly-growing fellowship. This was published as *Twelve Steps and Twelve Traditions*. It proposed to "broaden and deepen the understanding of the 12 Steps as first written in the earlier work".

"AA's 12 Steps are a group of principles... which, if practiced as a way of life, can expel the obsession to drink and enable the sufferer to become happily and usefully whole," its introduction explains.

"Though written mainly for members, it is thought by many of AA's friends that these pieces might arouse interest and find application outside AA itself," it continues.

"Many nonalcoholics report that as a result of the practice of AA's 12 Steps, they have been able to meet other difficulties of life... They see in them a way to a happy and effective living for many, alcoholic or not."

The 12 Steps now form the basis of self-help fellowships for people with different addictions and for their families, friends, employers and others close to them.

List of self-help fellowships. Sometimes called "mutual aid" groups, for example by the World Health Organisation, the following are some of those listed in *Addiction Today* journal, with contact details:

♥ ADULT CHILDREN OF ALCOHOLICS – www.adultchildren.org
♥ AL-ANON for families and friends of problem drinkers, including after they quit and ♥ ALATEEN for people aged 12-20 affected by someone else's drinking – for both 020-7403 0888 www.al-anonuk.org.uk
♥ ALCOHOLICS ANONYMOUS – 0845-7697 555 www.alcoholics-anonymous.org.uk
♥ CARERS ANONYMOUS for recovering codependents and addicts who care for someone with a mental and/or physical disability – www.carers-anonymous.org
♥ COCAINE ANONYMOUS – 0800-612 0225 www.cauk.org.uk

♥ CODA, Co-Dependents Anonymous –
www.codependents.org
♥ COSA for recovery from sexual codependency –
07986-697987   www.cosa-recovery.org
♥ DEBTORS ANONYMOUS – www.debtorsanonymous.org
♥ EMOTIONS ANONYMOUS – www.emotionsanonymous.org
♥ FAMILIES ANONYMOUS for relatives & friends of people
with drug problems – 0845-1200 660
020-7498 4680 www.famanon.org.uk
♥ FOOD ADDICTS IN RECOVERY ANONYMOUS, help with food
obsession, bulimia, overeating or undereating –
01903-520369   www.foodaddicts.org
♥ GAMBLERS ANONYMOUS plus
♥ GAM-ANON for relatives of problem gamblers
both: 020-7384 3040 www.gamblersanonymous.co.uk
♥ HEROIN ANONYMOUS – www.heroin-anonymous.org
♥ HIV ANONYMOUS – www.hivanonymous.org
♥ MARIJUANA ANONYMOUS –
07940-503438 www.marijuana-anonymous.org
♥ NARCOTICS ANONYMOUS for drug problems –
0300-999 1212 www.ukna.org
♥ NICOTINE ANONYMOUS – 020-7976 0076.
www.nicotine-anonymous.org
♥ OBSESSIVE EATERS ANONYMOUS –
www.obsessiveeatersanonymous.org
♥ OVEREATERS ANONYMOUS for problems with food,
including anorexia – 07000-784985
www.oagb.org.uk
♥ PAN FELLOWSHIP for any dependency/codependency
with emphasis on steps 4&10 – see *Addiction Today*
♥ S-ANON for people affected by someone else's sexual
behaviour – 07000-725463 www.sanon.org
cardiffhopefortoday@yahoo.com

♥ Sᴇx Aᴅᴅɪᴄᴛs Aɴᴏɴʏᴍᴏᴜs – London callback answer phone: 07000-725463 www.sauk.org
♥ Sᴇxᴀʜᴏʟɪᴄs Aɴᴏɴʏᴍᴏᴜs – 020-8946 2436
♥ Sᴇx & Lᴏᴠᴇ Aᴅᴅɪᴄᴛs Aɴᴏɴʏᴍᴏᴜs (The Augustine Fellowship) – 07951-815087 www.slaa.uk.org
♥ Sᴜʀᴠɪᴠᴏʀs ᴏꜰ ɪɴᴄᴇsᴛ ᴀɴᴏɴʏᴍᴏᴜs – www.siawso.org
♥ Wᴏʀᴋᴀʜᴏʟɪᴄs Aɴᴏɴʏᴍᴏᴜs – George 020-7498 5927 www.workaholics-anonymous.org

For any other issues, you can try www.ukselfhelp.info, a website containing hundreds of listings.

There are also specialist 12-Step fellowships for doctors (eg, The Doctors and Dentists Group), lawyers (eg, The Lawyers Support Group) and nurses. These are held separately to other groups mainly to ensure confidentiality, as people in these professions risk being struck off the professional registers – which should not happen when they are in clean and sober recovery, transforming their lives and helping others.

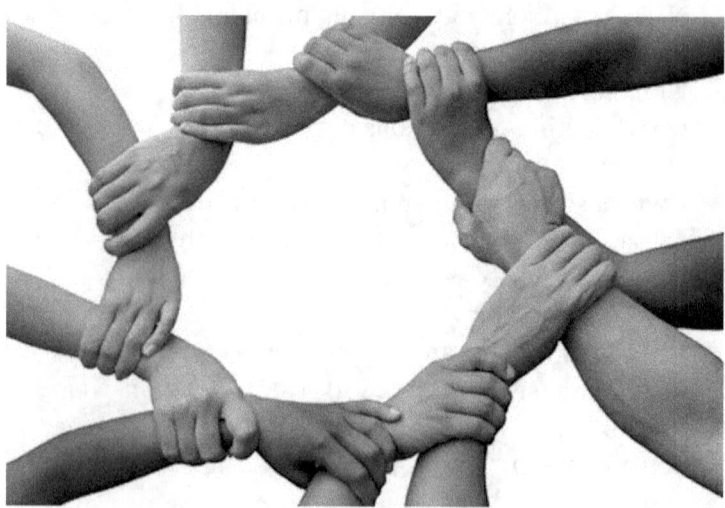

HOW IT WORKS

To write *The Twelve Steps*, the authors daringly consulted leading figures in the then-embryonic field of psychotherapy, including Carl Jung. So farsighted were the authors that anyone who today studies dynamic or integrative psychotherapy might be surprised to find that nothing in this 60-year old book contradicts their more recent learning.

People who want to recover from their addictions can get help from 12-Step meetings even before they apply the 12 Steps to their lives.

The first help, as the founders of AA discovered, comes from meeting people who have suffered or are suffering in a similar way. Most people who come to meetings believe that no one else is as bad as they are, no one else drinks/drugs/gambles/binges/behaves as badly they do, no one else lies about it and hides it like they do. To find that other people have been or are in identical situations immediately lifts some of the shame which prevents recovery. Newcomers are no longer alone.

To discover that not only have other people acted as inappropriately but that they miraculously no longer do so gives newcomers hope that they, too, can succeed like the solid, actual role models before their eyes. These people are not talking theory. They have lived the problem and have found the solution.

Going to meetings is also very practical in that it fills the time and the vacuum left by the addiction. When you are at a meeting, you cannot be in dangerous venues likely to lead to a relapse, or with users tempting you to do so.

If you say you are a newcomer, "oldtimers" will give you their telephone numbers for you to ring when you fear you might relapse. Do ring them. They are only doing for you what someone else did for them when they were new. This is their way of returning the favour. And, hopefully, when you are a few years in recovery, you will give your telephone number to newcomers.

Many people also go out for coffee and a chat after a meeting – "the meeting after a meeting". Merely by sitting and enjoying the chatter going on around you, you can learn that you can have fun and feel good about yourself without using an addiction.

In his bestseller book *The Road Less Travelled*, Dr Morgan Scott Peck defines the difference between a child's love and an adult's love, which I see as a description of how 12-Step fellowships work.

Scott defines a child as *being loved* until s/he is able to love. He defines an adult as *loving* until s/he is loved.

Newcomers are like children in their emotions when they come into a 12-Step fellowship. They are loved – in a caring, altruistic, *agape* sense – by longer-established members until they find their own capacity to love. Then, with their new-found emotional maturity, they can love newcomers who come after them.

It sounds idealistic. But it works extremely practically.

How fellowships work can also be explained by the therapist Abraham Maslow's list of the five hierarchical needs of all humans. These needs are called "hierarchical" because you cannot fulfill one need until the previous one has been fulfilled (exceptions are rare).

Maslow names the first need as physiological: warmth, food, water, shelter – and love. Experiments have shown that baby rhesus monkeys die when deprived of their mother's love. It is as necessary as all the other physiological needs.

Only when your physiological needs are secured can you meet the second need: safety. Many addictive people have never, as children or adults, gone past these two stages.

They have usually been deprived of love, through abuse or the death of a parent. They have usually been unsafe from adults who shamed them, ignored their needs, repressed their emotions, hit them or even sexually assaulted them. The 12-Step fellowship is probably the first time that they have felt loved and in the company of safe people.

Because of these earlier unmet needs, addictive people are unlikely to have reached the third hierarchy of needs: a sense of belonging and love. This is met, for many, again only when they are in the company of peers, people who have been through what they have been through.

As this diagram shows, the fourth level of need is for self-esteem, which has long eluded those who usually felt only shame before the benefits of recovery.

The fifth hierarchy is self-realisation, becoming "all that you can be".

These aims are not impossible if you work a good programme of recovery, as members of self-help groups have found in their own lives.

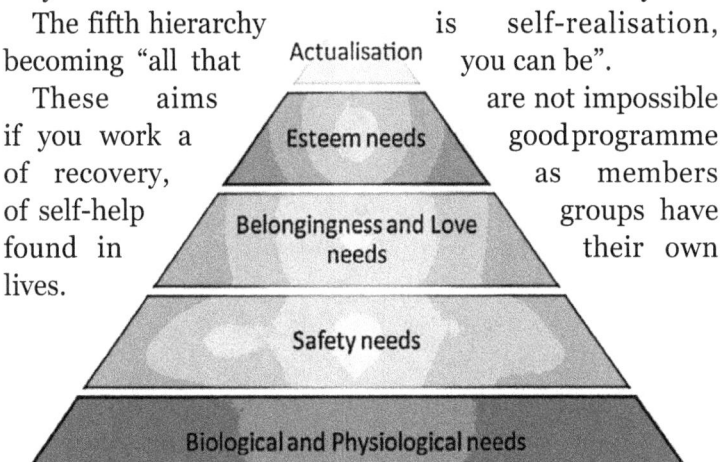

What can you expect when you go to a 12-Step meeting? First of all, you can make it easier on yourself by asking someone to go with you. Simply telephone the relevant "Anonymous" organisation and ask for someone to accompany you. This is regular service they offer, called 12-Stepping, so do not feel that you are asking special favours. Otherwise, ask someone you trust.

When you enter a meeting, there is usually a "greeter"

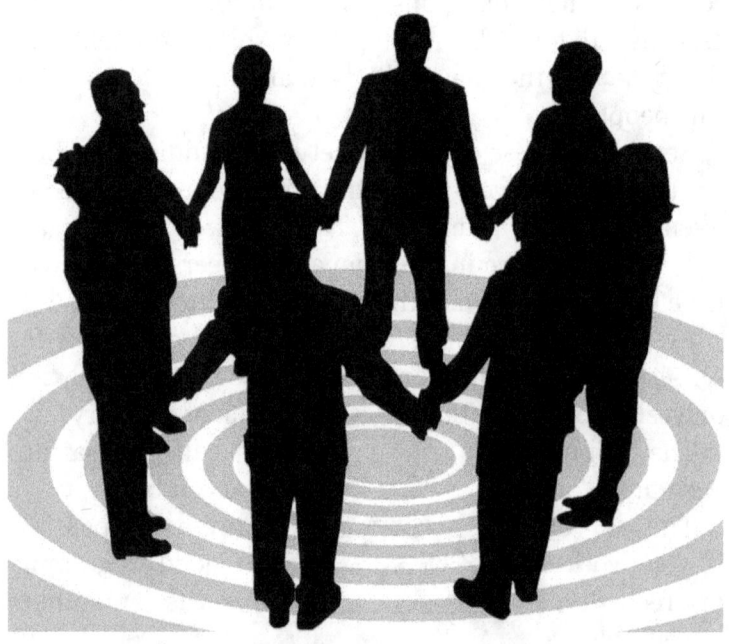

who will introduce you to a few people and give you a "starter pack" if you say that you are new to the fellowship. There is usually (free) tea and coffee, so that if you arrive early you can relax.

Meetings vary slightly in format and can last for an hour (if during lunchtime or rush hour) to an hour and a half (at other times). Usually, a "secretary" starts by briefly explaining the format, stating that the fellowship is open to all who have a desire to stop their addiction, that there are "no dues or fees" and asking for the 12 Steps to be read out. Then a "speaker" is introduced.

The speaker usually talks for 20-30 minutes. S/he tells her/his own story, what happened to them during their addiction, how they came to see that they had a problem, how they tried to stop it, how they found the fellowship, and what they learned and are learning in the fellowship to help them maintain their recovery and a happier, more fulfilling way of life. Sometimes the speaker will talk of the problems in their life and how they are trying to solve them without resorting to their old habits and addiction.

The rest of the meeting allows other members of the fellowship to "share" their own experiences. Sometimes they empathise with the speaker. Sometimes they have gone through similar problems and talk about the solution which worked for them. All this shared experience helps members to bond and to pick up positive feelings of hope and success. It emphasises the belongingness with peers.

Sometimes, 10 minutes of a meeting will be devoted to newcomers or people who find it hard to share. The more confident members will stay quiet so that they can do this. Take advantage of this when you first attend a meeting.

Just before the end of the meeting, a "pot" is passed around for voluntary contributions; put something in only if you can afford it. Then the "serenity prayer" is said (see Step 3 in this chapter).

The size of the meetings can vary from half a dozen to over 150 in popular central city areas. The members attending can be new and desperate for help or have been in recovery for decades. Some AA meetings are attended by people who have not drunk for over 40 years! They are often asked why they still go, to which they reply "it's because I go that I'm still sober".

Most people start going to meetings because they have to, but end up enjoying the companionship, help and support – a true fellowship.

You can also ask someone you trust in the fellowship to be your "sponsor". A sponsor is someone who agrees to help you with your recovery, particularly by guiding you through the 12 Steps. A sponsor is the person you can turn to first and most often when you are in difficulty.

Just one word of warning: there are some "oldtimers", usually men in their 50s, who know that newcomers are very vulnerable and have no scruples about borrowing money from them which will never be repaid or seducing them. It is hard to identify them because they usually speak well, and newcomers are susceptible – but you will come no harm provided you do not lend money or go to bed with an "oldtimer" in your first year. After that, you will be able to look after yourself.

Now, what are the 12 Steps and how can they help you to recover from your addiction? Below is a starting point.

THE TWELVE STEPS

1. "We admitted we were powerless over [name of addiction] – that our lives had become unmanageable."

The most important word of the 12 Steps is the first one: "we". The 12-Step fellowships work because people with similar histories meet to beat similar problems and to achieve recovery from addiction.

The first part of the sentence is the only part of all the Steps to refer to the addiction, or to stopping the addiction. The other 11 Steps refer to a way of life which helps you to stay stopped.

The first part of the sentence is also important in that it is only when you, or the person close to you with an addiction problem, "admits" that there is a problem that action can be taken to find a solution.

The second part of the sentence looks at the unmanageability which the addiction has brought into addicts' lives: unmanageable marriage and/or other unmanageable relationships, unmanageable or precarious work situations, compromised value systems, unmanageable feelings and reactions, unmanageable behaviour, missed and late appointments, unmanageable finances... the list goes on and on.

Looking at the damage which the addiction has caused provides a spur to staying out of the addiction.

2. "Came to believe that a Power greater than ourselves could restore us to sanity."

This sentence can be broken into many parts, starting from "came [to the meetings] to believe" and "came [eventually] to believe".

A "Power greater than ourselves" does not tie you down to any one religion or, indeed, any religion. It highlights that people used to make their addiction a power greater than themselves. Now you need a positive substitute, a substitute which protects your interests and health. You do not need to understand yet what that power is, just that there is something "out there" which cares more for you than you do for yourself, respects you more than you do, and is looking out for you.

For people who have problems with that, you can think of the people in your fellowship, with their experience and knowledge, as a power greater than yourself at this moment in time. Some people think of it as nature.

The 12-Step fellowships regard themselves as spiritual, which does not necessarily mean religious. One definition of spirituality is that it occurs when your emotional, physical and mental sides all work in sync. Another definition of the difference between religion and spirituality is that religion is for people who want to avoid hell – spirituality is for people who have been there. And all addicts know what hell has been like.

The last part of the sentence is "could restore us to sanity". One definition of insanity is "doing the same thing over and over again hoping to get a different result" — a good description of addictive behaviour, a definition by no less a genius than Albert Einstein.

Insanity is trying to avoid unavoidable reality through addiction. Insanity is worsening reality through your addiction. Insanity is cutting yourself off from feelings, being 100% "in your head" rather than your whole body. Insanity is pushing people away when you want someone close. Sanity is doing something different, something healthy. Sanity is coming to a 12-Step meeting. Sanity is changing destructive behaviour into constructive behaviour. Sanity is quitting addiction.

3. Made a decision to turn our will and our lives over to the care of God as we understood Him."

God, Power greater than ourselves, Higher Power... call it what you will, here we admit that our enormous willpower could not stop our addiction. Something else must come into the equation.

Step 3 says only that we made a decision, not that we actually managed to turn our will and our lives over to another power. All we need to do now is to make the decision. This show of willingness, of letting go of willpower, is the first of the "quality" steps, which bring relief, peace of mind and quality of life as we stop trying to control everything around us. What a relief.

The first two Steps help us to stop our addiction. From now on, we learn how living a quality life means that we have avenues other than addiction to keep us fulfilled. They can lead us up Maslow's hierarchy of needs to fulfilled lives.

The chapter on Step 3 in AA's *Twelve Steps* ends with "...it is really easy to begin the practice of Step 3. In all times of emotional disturbance or indecision, we can pause, ask for quiet, and in the stillness simply say

God grant me the
serenity to accept the things I cannot change
Courage to change the things I can
And wisdom to know the difference..."

4. "Made a searching and fearless moral inventory of ourselves."

There are only three, simple rules to know about Step 4: that you must put it in writing, that the only way you can get it wrong is by deliberately lying or deliberately omitting something, and that you leave as little time as possible between Step 4 and Step 5.

A fourth rule is related to Step 5 but it is now that you must think about it: choose someone to go through your Step 4 with you who can truly be trusted. This can be your sponsor – if you have not got one, find one for just this purpose – or even a therapist who understands the 12 Steps. Some people choose a priest, rabbi, or other holy person. It is your choice.

Step 4 is a list of assets and liabilities in our nature, the good and the worse parts of our behaviours. Writing down the liabilities means that we can recognise them and change them – sometimes, by the time we come to write our liabilities, we realise that we started changing some of them as soon as we came into recovery. Others take longer to change. This is often the first time we start to see ourselves as we really are.

I mentioned in Chapter 2 that, when I came into recovery, I was asked what kind of person I was. Was I mean or kind? Was I funloving? I could not answer.

It was not until I started writing my Step 4 that I could see what assets and liabilities were in my nature, and how often they cropped up. I started getting a picture of myself as a person rather than a work object.

When I wrote my first Step 4, I saw it as a test. My ideas about myself and my life had been validated so rarely that I did not know if my "answers" were correct. A year later, I did a second Step 4 (this is not obligatory) and felt a wonderful sense of humility even as I was writing: I was not the best in the world at being bad, nor the best at being good. I was ordinary – and so were my actions.

Even so, as I wrote out my assets I felt that I would be called a liar. Having my assets confirmed and validated was even rarer than having my reality validated.

Addictive people typically spend much time writing down their liabilities – but omit any mention of their assets. You must write down both to get a true picture. True humility is seeing yourself as you are, good and bad. Also, if you are overcome by all your defects you might feel too paralysed to move forward.

Take a break during your Step 4 if you feel tired or overcome by emotions. Telephone friends if anything you write makes you feel distressed. Telephone your sponsor. Start writing some assets. Finally, you can choose to do a bit of your Step 4, do a Step 5 on it, return to your Step 4, continue your Step 5, and so on.

"It is wise to write out our questions and answers. It will be an aid to clear thinking and honest appraisal," says the Twelve Steps. "It will be the first tangible evidence of our complete willingness to move forward."

I recommend Hazelden's excellent *Guide To Fourth Step Inventory* for people who want to take this Step.

5. "Admitted to God, to ourselves, and to another human being the exact nature of our wrongs."

"Scarcely any step is more necessary to long-time sobriety and peace of mind than this one," states the

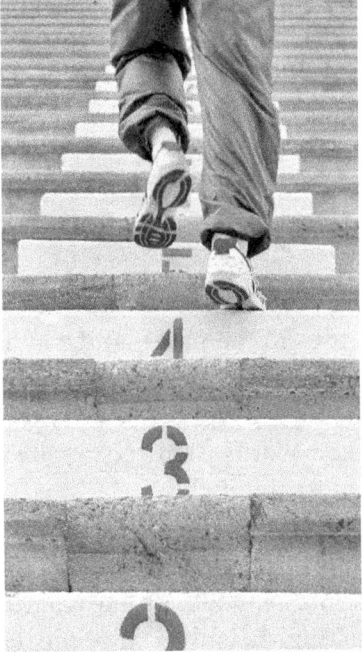

Twelve Steps. In Step 5 we go through what we have written in our Step 4 with someone we trust. For most addicts, this is the first time in their lives they have been validated. After sharing with the listener to their Step 4, they often hear that that person has done the things they have done – often worse. They are not isolated by their past actions. Deeds which they previously thought were too shameful to put into words are put into their small perspective.

Unuttered, they are a great amorphous fog; given a limited size on a piece of paper and compared to someone else's acts, they lose their power to instill fear and shame. They need no longer be drunk/drugged/eaten/gambled/relapsed on.

And as you describe your assets, you will find that your Step 5 listener believes in your assets more than you do! They will have already seen them but will not have dismissed or minimised them as you probably have.

Shame and guilt paralyse people, not only addicts. Step 5 lifts these two debilitating emotions so that you can move forward.

The practice of admitting defects to another person is ancient – before sponsors and counsellors there were priests. Psychiatrists and psychologists point out the deep need every human being has for practical insight and knowledge of themselves. It is no coincidence that addiction-treatment centres usually take their clients up to Step 5, before releasing them into the wider world to continue their development.

6. "Were entirely ready to have God remove all these defects of character."

In Steps 4 and 5, we identified our defects of character. Some of these have led to relapses in the past – and could do so again. Most have hurt us or others. Now we become willing to do something about them. We need not know what, just be willing. The key words "entirely ready" underline the fact that we want to aim high.

The *Twelve Steps* sums up this Step clearly. "Many will at once ask 'How can we accept the entire implication of Step 6? Why — that is perfection!'. This sounds like a hard question, but practically speaking, it isn't. Only Step 1, where we made the 100% admission we were powerless over [the addiction], can be practised with absolute perfection. The remaining 11 Steps state perfect ideals. They are goals toward which we look and the measuring sticks by which we estimate our progress. Seen in this light, Step 6 is still difficult, but not at all impossible. The only urgent thing is that we make a beginning, and keep trying."

Don't be daunted by the word "God": remember that the word can mean whatever you want it to be.

Finally, for some people, attending therapy is an ongoing Step 6 and Step 7 as they change what they do not like about themselves.

7. "Humbly asked Him to remove our shortcomings."

"Humbly" means with an understanding of both our assets and liabilities. It means seeing ourselves as we truly are. It does not mean humiliation, a word with which it is often confused.

Now that we can see ourselves much more clearly after Steps 4 and 5, and become willing in Step 6 to remove our defects, we lay a foundation for the future.

"Without some degree of humility, no alcoholic can stay sober," states the *Twelve Steps* clearly. "...But when we have taken a square look at some of these defects, have discussed them with another, and have become willing to have them removed, our thinking about humility commences to have a wider meaning. By this time in all probability we have gained some measure of release from our more devastating handicaps. We enjoy moments in which there is something like real peace of mind. To those of us who have hitherto known only excitement, depression or anxiety – in other words, to all of us – this new-found peace is a priceless gift... Where humility had formerly stood for a forced feeding on humble pie, it now begins to mean the nourishing ingredient which can give us serenity."

If the humility we used in Step 1 when we admitted we were powerless over our addiction was successful then, it can have a successful effect on our smaller defects.

8. "Made a list of all persons we had harmed, and became willing to make amends to them all."

"Steps 8 and 9 are concerned with personal relations. First, we take a look backward and try to discover where we have been at fault; next we make a vigorous attempt to repair the damage we have done; and third, having thus cleaned away the debris of the past, we consider how, with our new-found knowledge of ourselves, we may develop the best possible relations with every human being we know," promises the *Twelve Steps*.

Step 8 is writing a list of the people to whom you owe amends – bearing in mind that you probably owe more amends to yourself than to anyone else. To me, this is a grief list. List all your losses: not only deaths but also loss of relationships, friendships, jobs, money, and anything else which still disturbs you.

When you have finished, put an "R" or an "I" beside each entry. "R" stands for retrievable, "I" for irretrievable. You will be astonished to find how many things or people you had considered forever lost are still retrievable.

Don't act yet. Step 8 is only about making a list, not about acting. You might have stolen from people or hurt them in other ways when you were in the throes of your addiction. Now you need to list them – you might already have them in your grief list under loss of relationship with someone or loss of a job.

One good reason why Step 8 did not come earlier is that you need a clear head to know who you might owe an amend to and who you don't. For example, I had so little esteem in early recovery that, if I bumped into a door, I would apologise to it. It was the same with people: I assumed I was in the wrong about everything. I wasn't. When I wrote my list down, I found that I did not owe as many amends as I had expected.

"It is the beginning of the end of isolation," says the *Twelve Steps* about Step 8.

9. "Made direct amends to such people wherever possible, except when to do so would injure them or others."

The first thing to remember about Step 9 is that it comes after Step 8 – not after Step 1. You need everything you have gained from the first eight Steps in order to do Step 9 in a way that benefits your recovery.

The second thing to remember is that staying away from your addiction is the best amend you can make to yourself and to everyone close to you. The longer you stay away from your addiction, the greater the amend is.

The third thing is not to make any amend until you have the self-esteem to face its consequences; an amend is not about humiliating yourself.

The fourth thing is not to hope for a particular result from making the amend. There is no point, for example, returning stolen money to an employer in the hope of being re-employed. That is not what it is about; Step 9 is about restoring your conscience and peace of mind, so that you cannot relapse on your anxieties. Indeed, you will find that it is in many cases about restoring other people's peace of mind about you.

The fifth thing to remember is that an amend might not take the form you think. For example, stealing from a loved one cannot be atoned for by replacing the money. When you stole the money, you also stole their trust and peace of mind. These must be restored. You might have already gone a long way towards this by staying away from your addiction up to now, reassuring them that you can continue to stay away from it and the behaviours which accompanied it.

The final part of the Step states "except when to do so would injure them or others". If your partner, for example, is now enjoying a new-found peace of mind because of your recovery, do not shatter it by revealing past affairs with other people. You will then owe an even greater amend for this hurtful so-called amend. Damaging your relationship this way is also a trigger to relapse.

Finally, you might want to make an amend to someone but feel that it is impossible because they are dead or untraceable. Here, you can make a "proxy" amend, by making it to someone in as similar a situation as possible.

One woman I know, for example, wanted to make an amend to the child she terminated. Her amend was to look after vulnerable mothers with young children, an amend to both her past situation and that of her unborn child's. Other people write letters or poems to the dead, or carry out a specific wish they might have had.

10. "Continued to take personal inventory and when we were wrong promptly admitted it."

Step 10 is the only Step which gives a "quick fix". Say, for example, that you had an argument with someone close to you. Ask yourself: is it more important to be in the right or to retain the relationship? If you have been at fault, and can admit it to yourself, then a quick apology to the person with whom you have been arguing can save the relationship. If you are in the right, look at your situation in light of the boundaries in Chapter 5, guided by the "useful exercise before you say no".

Quickly admitting when you are wrong prevents relationships becoming adversarial. It allows you to move forward, forgetting the incident pretty promptly as a molehill has not been allowed to grow into a mountain.

Regular inventories can help save your recovery – resentment is a great prelude to a relapse.

One good idea in early recovery is to write down, just before you go to bed, all the pluses and minuses of the day – details of how you do this are in Chapter 6 under daily inventory. Some people take a more detailed inventory once a year or longer, to give themselves a spot-check and an overview of the progress they are making. This type of inventory has been called both a Step 10 and a Step 4.

Members of the Pan Fellowship centre their recoveries round these two steps.

11. "Sought through prayer and meditation to improve our conscious contact with God as we understood Him, praying only for knowledge of His will for us and the power to carry that out."

This sounds like the most "airy-fairy" of all the Steps, yet is the most practical. A half-hour's meditation at the start of the day can centre us for the rest of it. A walk or meditation in the park after an argument, or a holiday surrounded by nature can give us the objectivity to put things in perspective and inspire us with a solution.

This is about letting go after all your earlier footwork, about trusting and being 'in the moment'. "When we refuse air, light or food, the body suffers," the *Twelve Steps* explains. "When we turn away from meditation and prayer, we likewise deprive our minds, emotions and our intuitions of vitally needed support."

For people who do not like the idea of praying, it recommends the following start by someone who, although not known to be an addict, did go through the emotional wringer that all addicts do.

"Lord, make me a channel of thy peace – that where there is hatred, I may bring love – that where there is wrong, I may bring the spirit of forgiveness – that where there is discord, I may bring harmony – that where there is error, I may bring truth – that where there is doubt, I may bring faith – that where there is despair, I may bring hope – that where there are shadows, I may bring light – that where there is sadness, I may bring joy. Lord, grant that I may seek rather to comfort than to be comforted – to understand, than to be understood – to love, than to be loved. For it is by self-forgetting that one finds. It is by forgiving that one is forgiven."

St Francis of Assisi

"Perhaps one of the greatest rewards of meditation and prayer is the sense of belonging that comes to us. We no longer live in a completely hostile world," writes the *Twelve Steps*. "We are no longer lost and frightened and purposeless."

12. "Having had a spiritual awakening as the result of these steps, we tried to carry this message to [people with our addiction], and to practice these principles in all our affairs."

The "spiritual awakening" is the physical, emotional and mental awareness which comes to everyone who lives out a programme of recovery and stays away from their addiction.

"Carrying the message" is also known as "12 Stepping". It is when people who are in recovery help suffering addicts towards Step 1. It is adult love, as opposed to childish love, defined earlier in this chapter.

More formally, some fellowships allocate 12-Step rosters where members volunteer to be available to take a telephone call from an addict in need, to visit and talk to them, or to take them to a meeting. This is why newcomers should never feel afraid to ask for help: they are helping other members to fulfill their 12th Step.

Newcomers who think that a 12th Step is beyond them, can do it simply by coming to meetings. A successful meeting depends on at least two members turning up. Everyone at a meeting keeps everyone else coming. That is carrying the message.

"Practising these principles in all our affairs" means that we live the principles of this programme. The 12 Steps are not a theory or an intellectual opinion. They are a way of life which succeeds in keeping literally millions of people away from their damaging, deadly addictions.

"Our basic troubles are the same as everyone else's, but when an honest effort is made 'to practise these principles in all our affairs', well grounded [addicts] seem to have the ability... to take these troubles in stride and turn them into demonstrations of faith. We have seen [addicts] suffer lingering and fatal illness with little complaint, and often in good cheer. We have sometimes seen families broken apart by misunderstanding, tensions or actual infidelity, who are reunited by the [12 Step] way of life," explains the *Twelve Steps*.

The joy of good living is the theme of this last Step.

♥ ♥ ♥

If your personality does not suit 12-step groups, there are other self-help/mutual-aid groups described in *Circles of Recovery*, by Keith Humphreys who is currently drugs adviser to the White House.

8

How to change
someone you love

" *When someone we love, whom we want to help, says
no, it sounds like it is forever. It's not. It is a word at a
moment in time, not the end – and for many situations,
it will be the bridge to yes. This is key: we keep moving
forward in the face of a no. With or without agreement,
we continue making the change we seek...*

*"When I work with families, 'no' is just a conversation
starter. Behind that no is a yes dying to come out.* "

Brad Lamm, interventionist

In many ways, people close to an addict must 'let go' of
them, for everyone's benefit. But there is a right way to
try and initiate change before we let go. If your loved one
says no to coming to a meeting, to treatment, counselling
or other prescribed course of actions, there are several
strategies you can use. Perhaps the best guide I have
read is written by Brad Lamm: *How to change someone
you love: four steps to help* (details on page 152). The
practical tips in this chapter all come from him.

The advice in this chapter can also be used by therapists,
outreach experts and interventionists or given by them to
family members. Prepare yourself and your group ahead
to time to deploy them.

STRATEGY # 1

Use a technique designed to get a lesser commitment. Suppose you have asked someone to enter a 30-day inpatient addiction programme but he said "I will do anything you ask, but not that". Keep working for full agreement but if, after a couple of meetings, you remain stuck, consider compromise and a change agreement.

After the refusal, make a smaller request but one which is equally as helpful in motivating change. For example, you can propose: "Okay, I'd like to take you to a 12-step meeting. Why don't we start there? There's one today. Would you be agreeable to going there instead?". Or you could suggest "Okay, instead of six months of treatment, we could begin with 30 days?".

In many cases, he will view your second request as a concession, and feel inclined to respond with a concession of his own. This spot of concession and negotiation is often the first really tough spot you will have during the family meeting. Do not concede too early, as accepting help will often take some time. And you want a tangible change.

Seek to break through the no and get to the yes of full agreement before negotiating. By giving your love and care, you will most often get acceptance before you must negotiate. There is a very simple rule of human conduct at work here: the rule of reciprocity. It is a code which obligates people to repay what they have received. Reciprocity is a level of indebtedness.

Also, offering to attend the meeting with him carries weight. Knowing that you are there for him might make it easier. Typically, he will recognise that you are doing what any person who cares would do.

Another form of no is if she says "I can do this on my own". In response, tell her "We don't think that will work, but let's try your way for 30 days and see how things go". Of course, after the 30-day trial is up, and she has failed to get help, you meet with her again and ask her to go into treatment.

STRATEGY #2.

If you hear "no", take a break. Set a time to reconvene. Give everyone a chance to cool their heels and chat. Get together again and calmly restate the case for change. Reiterate the behaviours which concern you and your desire that your loved one gets help. Keep it simple. Stick with your major points and documented, observed behaviours of concern.

STRATEGY #3.

Try again. Schedule further family meetings and invite your loved one. Deliver updated change messages, Bring additional people into the 'circle of change'. There is no such thing as a failed family meeting. Each time you gather, you plant a seed. Your loved one might come back the next time and admit "Everything you say is true. I am ready to give it a go".

NO EVENTUALLY YIELDS TO YES.

Last summer, I worked with a family concerned about their daughter Lisa, who had an eating disorder. They held family meetings to get her into treatment. Lisa said no 43 times. I counted.

The mother of a little girl, Lisa's weight could be as light as 83 pounds. Her disordered eating took a toll not only on her body but also her family. They repeatedly urged her to get help, but she refused every time. The family never gave up. They kept repeating their central message: "What will your daughter do if something happens to you?" and "You need to be there for your daughter".

Finally, after five family meetings, that change message broke through. Lisa agreed to a compromise: seven days of intensive treatment at a disordered-eating clinic. The shorter treatment led to a full 42 days of treatment, where she finally began to fight her illness – and eventually won.

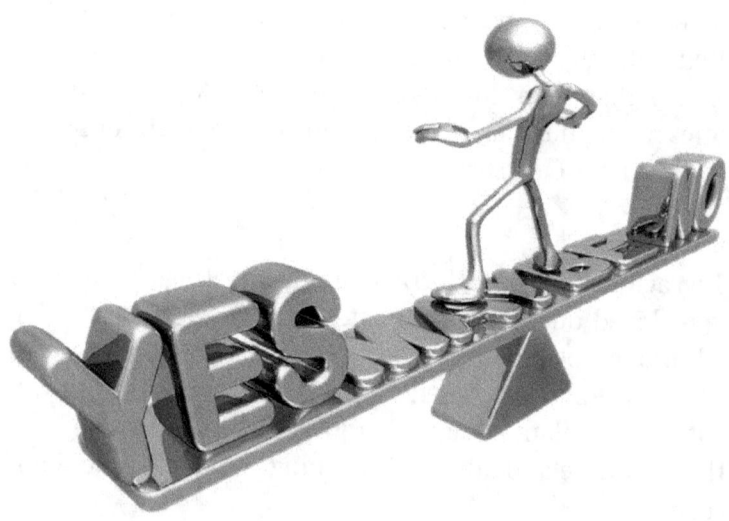

THE LEVERAGE STRATEGY: PLAN B

Do not give up if things do not go the way you want. Go to Plan B. I call this the leverage strategy. It sets up consequences of inaction. Yes, it is a little hard core, but it can be an effective motivator.

Money can be a great motivator when other things fail. Shelter. Food. Clothes. In other words, Plan B involves making use of consequences which help a person give change a chance.

I firmly believe we use only as much pressure as needed. But at times consequences are the way we help someone get unstuck from saying no. Saying that the "bank is closed: today we begin throwing our financial and other resources and energies behind recovery and change instead of the crisis" is a powerful statement which can be made when there is consensus built to back it up and stand firm.

You apply Plan B by spelling out consequences firmly but kindly. Here are some examples:

✗ We will no longer be able to give you financial assistance unless you enroll in counselling; we will support you but not your addiction

✗ Contact with the children or grandchildren will be cut off until you agree to go to treatment; we have a right to remove the children from destructive influences

✗ The police will be called when we fear for your – or our – safety

✗ You will have to move out until you get your anger/ behaviours under control

✗ We will no longer cover up for you

✗ You can no longer use the family car

✗ If you continue to resist change, you will lose your job

✗ Refusing to accept treatment means that we will have to separate or divorce.

Carefully prepared, structured consequences usually leave a person with more motivation to comply. A caution: do not bring up consequences unless you are willing to back them up. Usually, though, these situations are a last resort. Only 30% of the interventions I have done led to direct talk of consequences. The idea of consequences hangs in the air. Only make them real if needed.

Change will happen. You have as many tries as you wish to take.

Brad Lamm is a board-registered interventionist, founder of Intervention Specialists and author of *How to change someone you love: four steps to help* (available at www.bradlamm.com). Himself in recovery, he was a television news anchor and now focuses his TV work on family education.

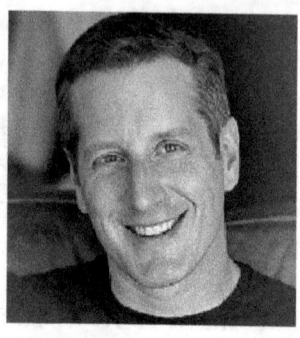

♥ ♥ ♥

9

Relapses and professional help

This chapter starts with the people who usually recognise the need for professional help first: the family affected by an addict's behaviour. At this stage, everything you have tried to get the addict to stop has failed, time and time again, cajoling or threatening. Attempts to get the addict to recognise their problem – far less do something about it – is usually met not only with denial of a problem but also anger, even rage. What can you do?

You can, of course, attend meetings for the families and friends of addicts (see Chapter 7) to help you cope with your feelings on a daily basis. You can try negotiation (see Chapter 8). You can also try a professional "intervention".

FAMILY / STRUCTURED INTERVENTIONS

This is a gathering of an addict's family, close friends – sometimes even employer – and possibly a professional "facilitator", usually seated in a circle, who try to persuade an addict that s/he has a problem and should seek treatment. Each person in turn starts by stating how much the addict means to him or her – but adds how damaged they have been by a *specific* behaviour or event caused by the addict. Addicts will usually not believe one person when they do not want to. But they cannot deny the cohesive opinions of many people, said not in anger but from love and a desire to help.

About nine out of 10 well-planned interventions succeed in getting the addict into recovery. Even interventions which do not persuade the addict to start recovery now plant important seeds for the future. They also give family members the feeling that at least they tried.

A successful intervention helps not only the addict but all others present, since they can finally tell the addict how they have been hurt by the disorder, and air their feelings and frustrations with a non-judgmental group to help make their case. Also, because the people present recognise the problem for what it is, they can take steps to help themselves.

Before setting up the intervention, ask everyone who will be there to write a list of specific events and behaviours which have caused them pain. The more ammunition of hard facts which you have, the more effective the intervention will be.

Older children and adolescents are usually very effective participants in an intervention. But do not bring in young children who will need to be cared for and distract you from the job in hand. Do not invite people whom you suspect might have an addiction problem of their own, as they could sabotage your efforts. And do not invite people who trigger anger in the addict, which could also sabotage your efforts.

It is usually best to ask a professional to facilitate the meeting, as they have the impartiality and experience to keep tempers down, to keep to the subject and not allow distractions, to keep things in perspective, to crystallise vague sentences and thoughts, to extract relevant information and to input specialist knowledge. Arrange a preliminary planning and education meeting with the professional, so that you are prepared as much as possible for the intervention. They will probably want to 'prep' all the people involved in the intervention.

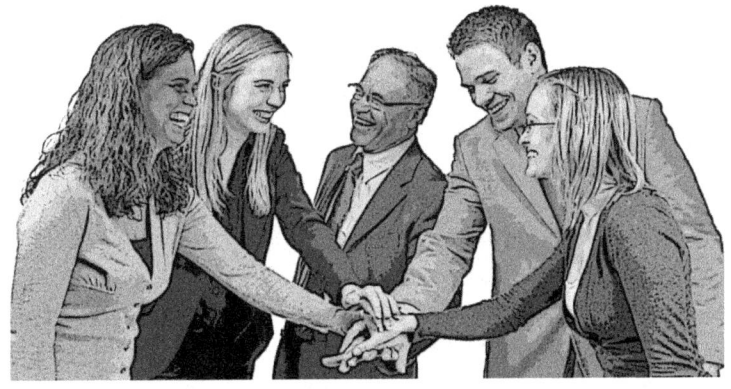

Further reading on interventions...

Two great books which describe interventions indepth and help you and the family to prepare one – there are even templates for letters to the addict, and behaviour contracts – are *How to change someone you love* by Brad Lamm (Chapter 8) and *Face It & Fix It* by Ken Seeley.

You can also read *Structured interventions: all you even wanted to know* at www.addictiontoday.org/addictiontoday/2009/10/structured-interventions.html

An extract about denial, from *Face If & Fix* It, can also be found at www.addictiontoday.org/addiction today/2010/04/face-it-fix-it.html

... and viewing

A&E TV's *Interventions* show is also excellent, offering the opportunity to view many real-life situations, so you can feel more confident about what is involved. You can view shows at www.aetv.com/intervention/index.jsp

AFTER THE INTERVENTION: TREATMENT

The facilitator or interventionist might agree to take the addict on for counselling, or might recommend another counsellor, counselling agency or a specialist treatment centre. Alternatively, you might like to read up on what is available by way of treatment centres first and choose for yourself. You can find lists and contact details in the US magazine *Professional Counselor* and the UK/european journal *Addiction Today* (www.addictiontoday.org).

Treatment centres often have waiting lists, so it is advisable to telephone the centre before the intervention, explain what you are doing, and synchronise the timing of the intervention with admission to treatment. If the intervention is successful, you do not want to waste an unique opportunity through unnecessary waiting.

If you do not have the funds for treatment, it is very difficult to get appropriate, effective care via government agencies – in the UK, less than 4% of those seeking treatment are referred to rehab. The Addiction Recovery Foundation charity has been striving to improve this, with Kathy Gyngell, Professor Neil McKeganey and David Best (see Introduction/Forewords). We trust that new policies in a new government allow more access to recovery.

Again, it is worth contacting treatment centres listed in *Addiction Today* for their advice about funding and any doctor or other person in a position to refer people into appropriate treatment. Most have excellent links.

If your or your loved one's problem is alcohol, and you have not managed to get treatment despite at least one crisis, it might also be worth contacting pressure group UK Advocates, founded by Bob Beckett, to help get a treatment place. Email info.soberlink@googlemail.com.

As an addict, if you have tried the recommendations in this book but still found yourself relapsing into your addictive behaviour despite your best intentions, you might have already realised that you need something extra, some professional help. This is no failure.

Sometimes there is something behind the addiction which only a professional is qualified to deal with. Sometimes you might be living with no support or with people who make life too difficult to handle alone. Sometimes you have not been given a manual to solve life's problems.

It might be that you do not need residential treatment, or prefer to see a private practitioner. It might be that you have to wait for treatment and a private therapist can keep you safe during the wait. Whatever your reasons, read the following guidelines before choosing a therapist.

Relapse-prevention specialists can ask their clients to commit themselves to six months' work on their recovery — a small slice of the rest of their lives. This could occupy an hour's session a week, or more.

They ask "What can you do to make it harder to relapse? How about turning off your money tap? Credit cards?". The suggestions come from the client: you.

Clients look at their contacts with alcohol/drugs/ addictive behaviour in their lives. They trace through pre-school, school and work areas on their psychological map. They look at childhood and adult friendships and relate them to addictive use.

Next comes a chart of their relapse sequences. Gerald Deutsch, a Cenaps-accredited [by Terry Gorski] relapse-prevention specialist, says that "this, in my experience, is a staggering encounter for clients".

Each relapse episode is then surveyed in closer detail. Tracing the history of a relapse is paramount to the solution. It is then we can identify the warning signs or "triggers" to relapse, be they external, internal or a combination. Now the client learns to manage those warning signs or triggers.

So the treatment runs its course: trigger identification, trigger management and recovery planning. The plan is evaluated from time to time by therapist and client. It takes in all aspects of your life: work, relationships, leisure activities, exercise, diet, health and fun – just as in Chapters 4-6 but with personal guidance.

Psychotherapist Martin Weegmann uses 'life maps' or 'recovery maps' to help clients identify their relapse triggers and the things which help them to stay clean and sober. The map on the right was by a heroin user – and it surprised him. Seeing what he was doing had a powerful effect, highlighting his immersion in drugs, and the users and dealers he could access. Indy added places like university and work which offered better prospects but were a struggle to reach.

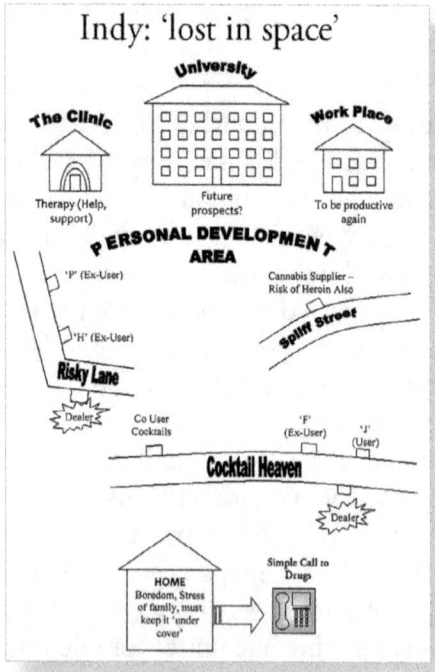

Indy: 'lost in space'

Drawing the map helped him to face his minimisation and denial. Five years on, Indy's map changed dramatically for the better. You can read more about Martin Weegmann's maps at www.addictiontoday.org/addictiontoday/2008/01/recovery-maps-g.html

There is no need, of course, for numerous relapses before seeking help from a counsellor/therapist for yourself or someone close to you. How do you choose? You do not go, as you might expect, to an institution representing "general" counsellors, some of which do not recognise addiction counselling!

Look for a counsellor accredited by IC&RC, the International Certification & Reciprocity Consortium. This sets the international 'gold standards' in addiction counselling, prevention, criminal justice, co-occurring disorders and clinical supervision through testing of addiction professionals. You can find more details, including local contacts, at www.icrcaoda.org.

In the US, you can also turn to a specialist organisation such as the National Association for Alcoholism and Drug Abuse Counselors: details at www.naadac.org.

In Ireland, you can go to the Irish Association of Alcohol and Addiction Counsellors (www.iaaac.org).

Surprisingly, in the UK it is hard to get a list of relevant addiction therapists. We are building one at the Addiction Recovery Foundation/*Addiction Today*. In the meantime, you can again telephone a treatment centre near you and ask them to recommend a specialist in your area.

Addiction counsellors and therapists tend to be in recovery themselves or have a family member in recovery. So they have both knowledge and experience of addiction and how to recover from it. Those who are in recovery are also invaluable role models: nothing inspires addicts looking for help more than someone who is living proof that you can be addicted and recover.

Ask if a potential counsellor is familiar with the 12 Steps, so that the counsellor supports you going to self-help support network between therapy sessions, and understands how they benefit you both. Look for someone else if they are not skilled in the 12 Steps.

Addicts also cannot as easily fool a counsellor in recovery with excuses: "you cannot con a conner", the saying goes. This is invaluable help.

The reason I do not advise a "general" counsellor or therapist at this stage is that many drink, drug, or use other addiction-prone behaviours in their own lives – recreationally or otherwise – and do not know how to treat people who must abstain totally. They also cannot provide an abstinence-free role model.

A "general" counsellor can be appropriate when you are established in recovery and need to deal with an issue in which they specialise. By then, you will have a solid background of addiction-recovery work and can afford to see a counsellor who will concentrate on something else. When I was almost six years in recovery, I started seeing such a counsellor because of the default post-traumatic stress disorder I was suffering from a *current* situation. This was outside the skills of most addiction counsellors.

Always look for an abstinence-based counsellor or therapist. Word-of-mouth is the best recommendation. And, if you have a choice, choose the counsellor or therapist who seems happiest with life, who has the emotions you want to have. If your counsellor can enjoy life without addiction, it augurs well for an enjoyable abstinent life for their clients.

The counselling provider – whether they are individual counsellors, in an agency of counsellors or a treatment centre – has an obligation to explain your rights and responsibilities to you, as follows.

A 'SERVICE USER' HAS THE RIGHT TO:

✓ Assessment of individual need, in a specified number of working days

✓ Access to specialist services, within a maximum waiting time (and immediate access on release from prison)

✓ Full information about treatment options and goals and involvement in making decisions about them

✓ An individual care plan and participation in the writing and reviewing of that care plan

✓ Respect for privacy, dignity and confidentiality, and an explanation of any exceptional circumstances in which information could be divulged to others

✓ Referral for a second opinion, in consultation with a GP, when referred to a consultant

✓ Development of service-user agreements, specifying the type of service to be delivered and quality

✓ An effective complaints system

✓ Information about self-help and advocacy groups.

A SERVICE-USER'S RESPONSIBILITIES TO THE SERVICE PROVIDER INCLUDE:

✓ Observing "house" rules and behavioural rules – for example, not using drugs on the premises, treating staff with dignity and respect, and observing equal opportunities and no-smoking policies

✓ Specific responsibilities in the framework of a care plan or treatment contract, such as keeping appointment times and observing medication regimes.

You might also wish to discuss in advance the choice of counsellor gender, where appropriate. For example, it is usually better to see a counsellor who is not of the same gender as the person(s) who maltreated the addict in the past, as this hinders the task of rebuilding trust. Ethnic-minority clients might want a counsellor who is culturally sensitive to their issues. So, too, might addicts struggling with gay/lesbian/bisexual/transgender/intersex and 'queer' or 'questioning' concerns.

Agencies also offer group counselling. This can start immediately or after you have learned to trust and share through individual sessions with a counsellor. When you go to an agency or counsellor, they will assess your needs, which type of counselling will suit you best and which counsellor is most appropriate for you. Their assessment will include whether individual or group counselling is most appropriate.

Group therapy usually consists of up to eight or 10 people, usually sitting in a circle so that you can all see each other, with one or two counsellors, called "facilitators" when they are in a group. This is to emphasise the fact that they facilitate, not run, the group. In other words, they encourage the members to interact with each other, and direct the group only when necessary.

It is decided in advance whether your group is closed or open-ended. In the former, it consists of a predetermined number of sessions, usually between six and 12. The same people start and finish the group together, and newcomers are not usually allowed to join. They might also centre round a specific subject matter.

An open-ended group can go on for an indefinite amount of time, can encompass a wide range of subjects, and might allow people to join in and drop out, so the profile of its members keeps changing.

The group consists of people who have had similar addictive problems. No one is worse or better than anyone else: you are all peers. You are about to discover together that you have similar solutions to those problems.

One member could start a group session by sharing a particular problem, either in the past or present. The facilitator usually asks if they would like feedback from other members about it. If agreed, the other members share their experience of similar problems and/or emotions, empathising with the first speaker. Others might have already found a solution and can share this.

Group therapy allows members to learn to bond with like-minded people. It helps them to form healthy

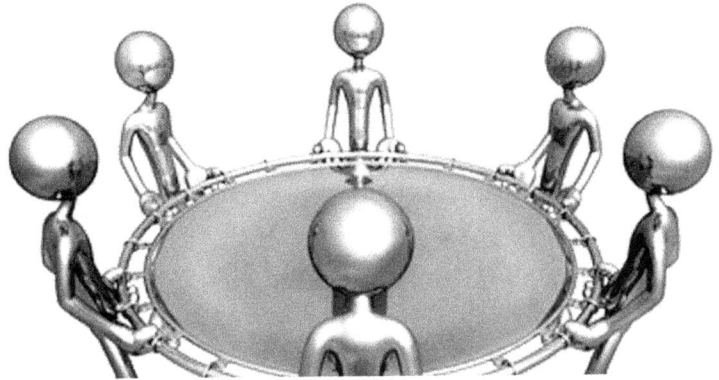

friendships. It helps them to open up honestly in front of other people. It removes the paralysing shame of past actions, as members learn that others present have done similar things. It helps members to see themselves more clearly as others feedback to them. And it helps them to confront others gently and with love. In short, it is a practice and a pattern for life outside the group.

First-stage residential treatment. Sometimes, an assessment might show that an addict needs to go into residential treatment rather than day treatment. Residential treatment is divided into two: first-stage and second-stage care, sometimes followed by third-stage which is lightly-monitored independent living. There are also "therapeutic communities" where the lines between the three stages are blurred.

First-stage residential treatment, often called "rehab", can last from four to eight weeks, depending on funding criteria, where you go and on the progress you make. Progress does not depend on intellectual strides: it is about accepting the damage caused by your addiction, and about getting in touch with your feelings.

First-stage units are usually mixed gender. Most work is done in group sessions, as already described. A mixture of psychotherapies is used, to give a holistic approach: getting your mind, body and emotions to work together. It is when clients get in touch with their feelings that they feel full with them. The emptiness, the vacuum, which had to be filled by anything – even dangerous addictive substances – is no more.

First-stage units based – sometimes loosely, sometimes tightly – on the person-centred Minnesota Model link their psychotherapeutic approaches to the first five of the 12 Steps described in Chapter 7, and ensure that residents attend 12-Step meetings during their stay. This is so that, when residents leave, they will feel comfortable in meetings and benefit from their ongoing support for as long as they like after leaving treatment.

More and more research shows that the vast majority of ex-residents who attend 12-Step meetings after treatment stay out of their addiction.

First-stage units can also offer yoga, meditation or other methods of relaxation where residents can learn to breathe properly and become more aware of their body. They are usually located in the countryside where you can go on walks in beautiful surroundings. This brings an element of spirituality into residents' consciousness.

Because of the intense internal work residents must do while in first-stage care, they are cocooned from the outside world so that it will not interfere. Here they truly learn the meaning of "keeping it in the day" for they are not allowed to look any further.

Residents usually finish with a Step 5, which allows them to move forward with a basis of self-knowledge, including identification of relapse triggers.

Second-stage treatment might be recommended when residents in first-stage care have nowhere safe to live after treatment. It can also be recommended if/when residents discover issues which must be investigated further before they can stay away from their addiction.

A mother can have so many demands made on her by her family, for example, that she needs to learn how to deal with them before she returns home. Someone else might fear that, if they returns to their live-in, drugging partner, they will relapse and needs time to come to informed decision and action about this. Someone else might have discovered childhood-abuse issues which leave them vulnerable to more abuse; they need time and protection while exploring these further.

You do not need to make any decision about this until you are about to leave first-stage care. This is just to reassure readers that there are more options open to them in the longer term.

Second-stage care is less intense than first-stage. There might be one group therapy session a day rather than three – there might even be only one session a week. There is at least one individual counselling session a week. Again, most units recommend that residents attend 12-Step meetings so that there will be ongoing support when they leave.

This is where residents learn to grab hold of their lives again. From a safe distance, they prepare themselves and their home, work or other situations for their return. There is much emphasis on boundaries and how they should be used in their individual home and work situations. Life skills can be taught, including training for a career. Where first-stage care has given a blueprint for the future, second-stage lays deep foundations on which to build whatever you like.

Involving families in treatment. Research also shows that the most powerful predictor of whether a client will complete treatment is their family involvement. Involving the family also helps ensure that the addict returns to an environment which encourages recovery and discourages addictive behaviours. And it helps the family members themselves...

"A family is a place where minds come in contact with one another. If these minds love one another the home will be as beautiful as a flower garden. But if these minds get out of harmony with one another it is like a storm that plays havoc with the garden," Buddha said.

To create that harmony, almost all rehabs offer a "family day", usually at the weekend, or a weekday evening. Others offer a "family week" where families can work with professionals on their concerns before safely meeting again with the addict, who has simultaneously been working on his/her issues. These family members also share time with families of other patients: peers with whom they can share tribulations, lessons and successes.

PREDICTORS OF SUCCESS

There are no guaranteed predictors of successful recovery through treatment. However, the first edition of this book featured research by Broadreach House which has since been consolidated by other research projects. Broadreach had commissioned an independent researcher to assess its files of over 2,000 clients to see which denominators were common to clients who successfully completed treatment, which is an indicator of long-term recovery. The results were as follows:

1: The most powerful predictor of whether a client will complete treatment is their family involvement, no matter how little
2: The higher the status of the client's most recent employment, the better the outcome
3: Female clients are more likely to complete (probably due to the fact that female counsellors tend to be more successful)
4: Alcoholics are more likely to complete treatment than users of other drugs (this might be due to their better socio-economic factors)
5: The more years the client has been addicted, the better the outcome
6: The shorter the wait to get into treatment once decided, the more likely the client is to complete treatment
7: Previous contact with a self-help group – a little exposure is better than a lot, which is better than none.

As mentioned, readers can get a list of treatment centres in the *Addiction Today* journal or going to the www.addictiontoday.org website and clicking on the "Treatment Centres" tab near the top of the homepage. US readers can get a list from *Counselor* magazine at www.counselormagazine.com.

The next two chapters look at treatment for specialist groups: adolescents, people forced into treatment, with other mental disorders or with physical disabilities.

♥ ♥ ♥

10

Special cases:
children, adolescents

" *Who so neglects learning in his youth,*
Loses the past and is dead for the future. **"** Euripedes

" *Drug abuse can damage a child's ability to go to*
school, to succeed and to live a normal life. At worst,
substance abuse can ruin a child's life. At best it can limit
their ability to learn and succeed. Use of drugs also
affects their family, friends and everyone in their life. **"**
Home Office

Any parents who want to do their best to prevent their
children from developing alcohol and other drug problems
must make a conscious effort to learn four things:
- How to communicate with their children
- How to let their children express their feelings
- Boundaries, and
- Knowledge about addiction.

By reading all the chapters so far in this book, you will
have made great inroads into the last two of the above.
By learning to express your own feelings through the
previous chapters, you will also have made great strides in
allowing your children to express theirs similarly. So we
come to communicating with your child, something which
cannot start too early.

You might also need some knowledge about specific drugs with which your children's peer group are experimenting. Pamphlets and web advice are widely available, such as from the UK government's Home Office (http://drugs.homeoffice.gov.uk/young-people) and at the US government's National Clearinghouse for Alcohol and Drug Information (http://ncadi.samhsa.gov).

Also, a heavily-evidenced *Parents' Resource Manual* reviews international research to identify best practice in prevention of substance use – download it free of charge from *www.drugsandalcohol.ie/12336/1/parents_manual_literature_review.pdf*. Part 2 of this will identify current programmes, strategies, interventions and resources for parents.

PREVENTION

It had been thought that the australian government led the way in drugs- and alcohol-prevention programmes for children, as it pioneered information about these on the school curriculum. But, seemingly against all logic, surveys increasingly show that this accelerated drug experimentation in children. At best, it made children aware of drugs but did not change their behaviours towards drugs.

What we have learned is that how we communicate information is vital. "Scare tactics" do not work. A recovering addict who visits schools to talk about their addiction and recovery has more credibility with schoolchildren than a didactic lecturer – even more so when that recovering addict is about the same age. One handsome recoverer takes out his teeth with great effect to show how they decayed through drug use!

Teenagers and young children today are faced with major challenges which leave them vulnerable to addiction and which did not exist in their parents' school days: the wide availability of mood-altering substances, peer pressure to be "accepted" by using these, lower educational standards, peer pressure to be accepted by getting a girl/boyfriend as early as puberty, family separations and "blended" families when both parents take new partners. As ever, there are also family conflicts, and addicted or dysfunctional parent(s) with all the consequent damage to their children.

Parents need to prepare for adolescence, to be aware that their child is about to form a more autonomous personality and bridge the gap between childhood and adulthood. One international expert in this area is Dr Kathy Hirsch PhD, a clinical psychologist who specialises in child, adolescent and family development. She is director of cognitive-behavioral therapy at Familyhealth Associates (http://familyhealthassociates.info). The following information in this section comes from her experience; it has not aged since the first edition of this book...

Adolescents experience psychological changes as well as the obvious physical ones. One US survey showed that parents who were unprepared for this suffered a mental-health deterioration as a result! So let's prepare.

As the children go through puberty and adolescence, self-esteem becomes pre-eminent in shaping their future lives. Self-esteem is shaped here by three factors: appearance, popularity and intelligence. People's body image is usually formed in adolescence and will stay with them through their lives. If they think they are fat, they will always see themselves as fat, no matter how slim they are; you can see the potential for anorexia or bulimia here.

Popularity depends on their peer group. If they feel inadequate, they can act out by, for example, playing the clown or using drugs and alcohol. If the acting-out gives them a more "successful" image with their peer group, they will continue to do it.

If you think that your child is acting out, you need to identify and address the issues they are struggling with – such as feeling unintelligent at school – to understand and address the behaviour.

A child's peer group forms part of his/her identity. Children aged 12 to 13 years old are most susceptible to outside influences such as this. Find out why a particular peer group attracts your child, so that you can encourage or discourage them from its influence.

These children are learning new socialisation skills, how to form interpersonal relationships. Parents see it as losing power, that their children are abandoning the values they taught them. Do not panic. Peer-group influence falls away from its peak of 12- to 13-years old. Parental influence continues into adulthood. Children are not separating from their parents. They are becoming connected in a new way.

At this time, parents feel unable to communicate with their growing children – while teenagers feel the same way about their parents.

How do you like people to respond to you when you are upset? Adolescents need the same consideration. If you cannot express your feelings, you will feel awkward allowing your children to express theirs.

Seven parental modes which close off communication with their children rather than opening it up were identified by Don Dinkmeyer and Gary McKay in *The Paents' Handbook*. They are described opposite.

How parents close off communication
with their children:

✗ COMMANDER-IN-CHIEF – typical phrases include "shape
up", "pull yourself together" and "set a good example";
it is all about control, not about allowing the child to
express what is going on

✗ MORALIST – typical phrases include "should", "should
not" and orders to the child to have "proper" or "good"
feelings with which the adult is comfortable. This again
dismisses the child's feelings and closes the
conversation. After this, how can you bring up more
important issues such as addiction?

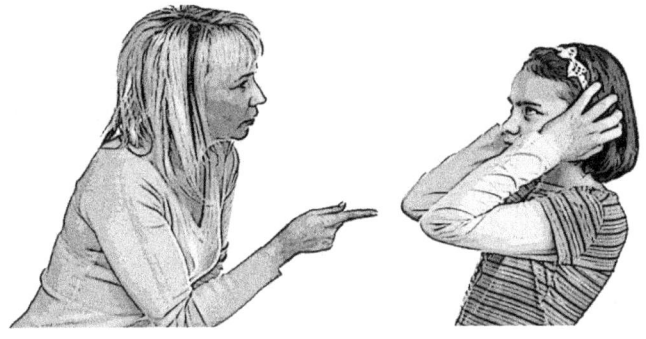

✗ KNOW-IT-ALL – the parent lectures, appeals to reason,
shows that they are superior to the child

✗ JUDGE – finds the child "guilty" without a trial; the
parent is always right, the child is always wrong

✗ CRITIC – ridicules, name-calls, uses sarcasm and jokes.

✗ Psychologist – tries to analyse the feelings away, rather
than allowing them just to be

✗ CONSOLER – excuses themselves from involvement by
treating emotions lightly; gives a pat on the back
and says the "worries will disappear" or "there are
other children a lot worse off than you".

How can you expect your children to suddenly open up about drugs or other addictions when their experience has been that you have shut them off, as on the previous page? As soon as you change your attitude, you have started your addiction-prevention work.

Basis for communicating with your children

- ♥ AIM: MUTUAL RESPECT. Express yourself honestly without fear of rejection and allow your child to do the same. You might argue with what your child is saying, but you must acknowledge the feelings.
- ♥ LISTEN. Listen with your eyes by maintaining eye contact.
- ♥ CONCENTRATE. Use body language which says "I am listening", such as leaning forward, facing the child.
- ♥ OBSERVE nonverbal forms of communication: facial expressions, body language, tone of voice, general appearance, how they respond to others, attitude, who sits next to whom.
- ♥ VALIDATE: let them know that you have heard them. Reflect and clarify their feelings. Restate them so that your child feels accepted. For example, your child might come home one day complaining that "My teacher is unfair; I'll never do well". Your reply could be "You feel angry and disappointed; you have given up". You have now opened up the communication.
- ♥ FEEDBACK. You have listened to, clarified and validated. Repeat this with your child's next response (this is called feedback).
- ♥ EDUCATE. Give basic information about addiction and codependency in a way your child can understand. Help them to realise that any family problems are not their fault; introduce them to healthy living skills,

including identification and expression of feelings, problem solving, self-care strategies, and exercises building self-worth.

- EMPOWER. Help children to identify safe people to whom they can turn for support and guidance. Help them to realise they are not alone.
- OPEN V CLOSED RESPONSES. In a closed response, the child does not feel heard or understood. You might feel that you have responded but have cut the lines of communication – refer to the seven parental modes. An open response reflects the speaker's message and allows the communication to expand.
- FINALLY, LISTEN AND REFLECT BEFORE REACTING. Let your children learn. Resist the impulse to impose your own solutions. As children become adolescents, they must still have rules but guidance and feedback replace demands and directives.

Adolescence is a smoother ride for parents who can remain active and involved with their teenagers. They need an authoritative but not authoritarian approach. Teenagers need to feel that they have contributed to the rules. So agree a "family set of rules" in which children have some input but the parents make the ultimate decision. They are then more likely to keep those rules.

This is where boundaries come in (Chapter 5). Children need to learn that breaking rules has consequences. Using drugs including alcohol and tobacco come under this heading. Discuss them along with other rules, not as a particular subject in itself.

Why are children attracted to drugs? Why do they experiment? Responses from Dr Hirsch's clients include:

"I feel invincible"   "It feels good"
"It's hard to say no to my friends"   "I feel like an adult"
"It relaxes me"   "It's fun"
"To be accepted by my friends"   "To escape".

The response from children who do not use drugs is "fear of disappointing my parents". Their response to being asked the difference between them and their friends who do use drugs is "I talk to my parents". Your open communication is vital in trying to prevent addiction.

Summary of addiction-prevention measures:

1. Start talking early, and keep talking
2. Look for timely moments when your children are receptive, but do not wait forever
3. Listen to your children; reflect and clarify what they say
4. Build a "community check" with other parents (for example, if your child tells you that "everyone" is going to a certain party, check with other parents)
5. Teach your children how to express their feelings
6. Do not threaten; it only lowers credibility
7. Roleplay situations such as peers offering drugs, being drunk, etc
8. Respect your children's behaviour when they say "no" and become independent
9. Praise your children when they are right and do well
10. Give them positive labels; for example, refer to their "mature" behaviour
11. Develop common interests: go to community events, sporting events, plays and films with your children.
12. Be a good role model – children do as their parents do, not as their parents say!

Warning signs of teenage substance abuse:

Fall in school work	Rebellious behaviour
Withdrawal from others	Isolation
Chronic fatigue/lethargy	Change in friends

Loss of interest in hobbies/sports
Change in relationship with parents
Chronic lying about whereabouts
Sudden disappearance of valuables and money at home
Mood changes with no discernible cause
Abusive behaviour to self and others
Outbursts of hostility without understanding why
Chronic dry, irritating cough/sore throat
Chronic conjunctivitis otherwise unexplained.

It might come as a surprise to learn that the period between 3pm to 6pm is when adolescents are most likely to succumb to alcohol, drugs or sex. This is because they are likely to be unsupervised as school has finished but their parents are not yet back from work.

You have found drugs/alcohol in your child's room – what to you do?

✓ Do not panic
✓ Do not shout
✓ Wait 24 hours before saying anything and work out carefully what you want to say
✓ Speak to a trusted friend, get feedback, go for help
✓ Talk to your child
✓ Gather information: who, what, when, where, why
✓ Punishment is best in the form of restricting privileges, such as use of the telephone. Give your child the power to redeem him/herself by earning privileges back. Teach your child there is are consequences to actions.
✓ Seek professional help.

CHILDREN FROM HIGH-RISK FAMILIES

Children who come from families in which addiction already exists are particularly vulnerable to becoming addicted themselves. One professional who specialises in prevention/intervention for children in high-stress, high-risk families is Jerry Moe, children's programme director at the Betty Ford Center.

"The first concept for children to learn is that addiction and codependency are a family disease. Everyone in the family gets hurt by it," he says. "The other two key concepts are for the children to accept that family addiction and

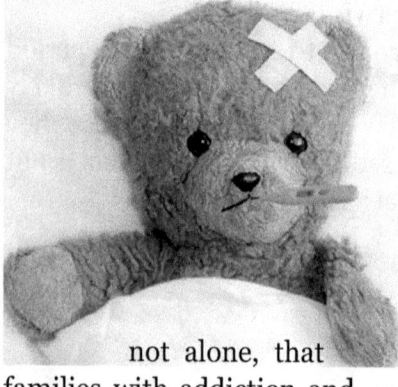

codependency are not their fault, and that they are themselves at high risk for addiction and codependency."

He instills the three key concepts into the children, and helps them to realise they are not alone, that many children live in families with addiction and codependency.

The first day of his programme is called "not my fault", and is about family addiction and codependency. The second day is "all my feelings are OK". The third is "taking care of me" which is about problem solving and self-care. And the fourth is "I am special", developing self-worth.

He has produced a workbook which can be used by parents, teachers and therapists – *Discovery: Finding The Buried Treasure* – which has exercises you can work through with children from as young as four years old right through their childhood.

ABUSE vs ADDICTION

Some parents condone teenage use of alcohol and even "recreational" drugs. But mood-altering substances will delay their development. More importantly, there could be life-long consequences due to irresponsible behaviours while under the influence. Joy-riding while drinking, getting pregnant or a sexual disease including HIV, and death from Ecstasy are some which spring to mind.

It can be hard to distinguish between abuse and addiction in teenagers, as they do not have enough substance-abuse history to make a definitive diagnosis. It can help to look for the following characteristics, identified by Tammy Bell who has been working with adolescents since 1981. A lecturer and consultant, she is director of relapse-prevention services for the Cenaps (www.cenaps.com/The_Cenaps_Corporation/North_Carolina.html).

◇ evidence of tolerance and withdrawal (see Chapter 2)
◇ mental preoccupation and craving; preoccupation includes thoughts of procurement, planning, actual use, euphoric recall and recovering from the effects
◇ how strong is the desire to use?
◇ what is the teenager willing to go through to do it?
◇ what is s/he willing to give up to use?
◇ how has substance use affected his/her interest in other areas of life?
◇ loss of control
◇ unable to stop, despite the consequences
◇ tries to change circumstance, not substance use
◇ is there a genetic predisposition?

It is important to spot the difference as early as possible, to organise the appropriate treatment.

Bell cites the paramount importance of peer groups. Adults, no matter how much they have in common with adolescents through their addiction, are no substitute for an age-appropriate peer group. So self-help meetings packed with adults and adult-oriented treatment are not attractive to adolescents.

To get around the first, Bell recommends that you ask an AA/NA member to escort an adolescent to their first few meetings. Recruit a temporary sponsor to mentor them for four to six weeks. This temporary sponsor can attend meetings with the adolescent, have post-meeting discussions to understand confusing concepts, and help relate the concepts to the adolescent's peer group, school, parents and others.

TECHNIQUES FOR PEOPLE "FORCED" INTO TREATMENT

To get round the aversion to adult-oriented treatment, Bell has run six-session weekly outpatient "pre-treatment" or "motivate-toward-recovery" programmes. These can also be used for people ordered by a court of law to get treatment and others "forced" into treatment. It has three overriding themes:

1: connecting life consequences to drug/alcohol use
2: giving up the belief that they can control their drug/ alcohol use
3: controlled abstinence.

For the first, a peer group of adolescents are encouraged to "brainstorm" their current problems and list them on a flipchart; 10 to 14 is a good number. Until now, adolescents believe that their lives are normal and their life problems have nothing to do with their alcohol or drug use. They feel that "hysterical" or "over-reacting" adults are forcing them into treatment. They have not had time to evaluate their use.

Bell does not mention mood-altering substances at this stage. Instead, all she asks is that the clients study the list and see if they can work out the cause of the problems.

In the second session, she takes the list of problems back up and gets a new flipchart sheet headed "Causes". It is impossible for chemicals not to come up over and over again – but suggested by the clients, not Bell. The homework is simply to solve the problem.

When connecting life problems, find out which are important to the clients – for example being kicked out of school might not be, but getting a girlfriend back is!

Almost all the clients come back to the third lesson suggesting that they should "cut down" their use. If the adolescent is a social user, this will work. If not, you probably have an addict on your hands.

Adolescents – like many adults – need to try control before abstinence. We must respect that, but without encouraging use of mood-altering chemicals. Adolescents need to put their belief systems through the experience about which chemicals they can get away with.

Adolescents must make this discovery for themselves, so that they are more highly motivated to do something about it. If you point it out to them, they will counter-react. This way, the first light goes on, followed by a reluctant, small admission. This is much more motivational than any lecture on addiction or behaviour.

Bell warns people not to build in rewards for compliant clients or punish those who are truthful about relapsing. The latter are the better client in that they are consciously experiencing the consequences of abusing chemicals.

At this stage, she and the client draw up together a plan of action "now that we know you cannot control your drug". They might suggest abstaining for a limited period, perhaps to prove something to a judge or parent. As they leave a session with her and before they try, Bell extracts a promise. "I think you can do it. But just perhaps, maybe, you can't, will you promise to do something for me? In the unlikely event that you fail, will you try a treatment programme?" The clients promise because they are positive that they will not fail.

Now we move into the third and final phase: controlled abstinence. These clients do not make lifestyle changes. They continue going to raves where friends take drugs, for example. Adolescents have not yet learned to delay gratification and are ruled by impulses. They are also immersed in a drugs subculture. It will take time for them to learn that they must leave using-friends behind.

Family intervention is the final thing which Bell uses. She also recommends a "vibrant, vital" role model aged between 16 and 18 years, with street credibility, to talk to the adolescents about their own recovery. When she first started working with adolescents and could not find someone in recovery of their own age, a recovering 28-year old biker gave a successful talk. "Kids like funky."

When taking someone through pretreatment, three major goals are accomplished. There is a thorough assessment over the six to eight weeks of sessions. It allows the clients to work through pretreatment tasks. And it allows motivational counselling, so people are motivated towards recovery.

One final reminder about trying to prevent addiction and maintain recovery: Children will do as you do, not as you say. You must be a reliable role model.

Special cases: 'dual diagnosis'

> **"** *Wine drunk with equal quantities of water puts away anxiety and terrors.* **"**
>
> Hippocrates

Hippocrates was right: wine and other drugs can mask mental unease. Some people recover from addiction – then find that they have diagnosable depression or schizophrenia which has been masked by their drinking or drugging. Others might have difficulty getting clean or sober, or constantly relapse, because they have a psychiatric disorder entwined with their chemical dependency. People who have both a chemical dependency and another psychiatric illness are described as having a "dual disorder", "co-occurring disorder", "dual diagnosis" or "comorbidity". They tend, perhaps understandably, to self-medicate their pain.

Included under the heading of dual diagnosis are people whose even occasional use of alcohol or drugs causes problems serious enough to warrant treatment. For example, schizophrenics who take marijuana will likely forget to take their daily medication which keeps their lives manageable; they can then relapse back into the mental-health disorder with all the pain and suffering it causes not only them but all their family. This link has been evidenced in some cases of killings by schizophrenics.

Studies indicate that drug or alcohol problems hamper the recovery of up to 75% of psychiatric patients. So if someone close to you has been having constant psychiatric problems, look at their alcohol/drug use. It might give you new hope for recovery from the mental disorder, alongside recovery from the substance use.

For example, people with depression might find that it was completely due to alcohol – which they had thought eased the depression. People whose depression is 'organic', due to chemicals and processes sitting in the brain near those affecting addiction, can find that the self-help techniques for recovery from addiction also ease their symptoms.

In 1990-1992, the National Institute of Mental Health published the first US comorbidity survey, which is an international benchmark (there are no comparable figures in the UK). With over 20,000 adult participants, it found that 37% of alcoholics had a mental disorder, and 53% of drug addicts/dependents had at least one psychiatric disorder, as did 64% of drug abusers in treatment.

So it is worth reading more information about this.

The most common dual disorders are: bipolarity and schizophrenia (affecting more men than women) and depression (affecting more women than men). The other most common dual disorders are personality and anxiety disorders. All are briefly described in this chapter

The statistics are not as gloomy as they at first appear. For example, most substance-induced depressions disappear within a few weeks of abstinence.

As well as depression, using or withdrawing from mood-altering chemicals can result in mania, anxiety, panic, paranoia, delusions and hallucinations. For example, hallucinogen or stimulant users can become psychotic and appear schizophrenic. People who abuse tranquillisers can show agitation and anxiety symptoms when they cut back or stop using them. Deal with the addiction, and these troubles can disappear.

12-Step programmes (as in Chapter 7) emphasise the role of personality-change in the recovery process. Steps 4, 5, 6, 7, 10 and 12 in particular are about changing "character defects", useful in dealing with personality disorders.

It is my experience that people who live a thorough programme of recovery from addiction, including counselling with the right therapist for them, deal with many mental disorders – without putting a psychiatric label on them – as they deal with their addictive way of life.

Cutting, dependency disorders, antisocial disorders, chronic stress disorders including post-traumatic stress disorder and borderline personality disorders, and other effects of childhood abuse... these are only some issues which I know to have been effectively dealt with in counselling for addiction recovery. This is why you must choose your counsellor carefully.

A *caveat* here: while people with neurotic disorders respond very well to the same therapies which apply to recovery from addiction, people with psychotic disorders usually require medication in order to stabilise first – therapy might be wasted or need to differ.

People with dual disorders are more likely to relapse than people without. Therapy must address both conditions.

The suggestions for recovery in this book work not only for addiction but also many dual disorders. Indeed, they are an excellent self-help tool if you have one of the disorders mentioned earlier, even without the addiction!

It must be stressed again, however, that therapy sometimes does not hold all the answers. Some people need psychiatric help and specialised medication.

Further reading. Because dual disorders is a relatively new area even for the professionals, you should read up on the subject if you suspect that you or someone close to you has a dual diagnosis. If you want more information, there is an excellent choice of inexpensive pamphlets and books on general and specific dual disorders from Hazelden, including *Addiction and Mood Disorders: A Guide for Clients and Families* by Dennis Daley with Antoine Douaihy. You can also read more at the helpful website www.helpguide.org/mental/dual_diagnosis.htm.

What is obvious as you read the symptoms of the mental disorders in this chapter is that they are similar to people's traits when they are in active addiction. It is only when people stay out of their addiction that you can clearly see whether the symptoms really do belong to a mental disorder or whether they disappear with the addiction.

In other words, if you or someone close to you exhibits the following symptoms, do not suspect a mental disorder unless they continue after a period of abstinence.

All the symptoms listed in this chapter comply with the American Psychiatric Association's *DSM-IV*. They apply only when the traits are NOT due to drugs/medication, a medical condition or another psychiatric condition. All traits must be inflexible and persistent, impair functioning or cause subjective distress.

Major depression and dysthymia. "Major" is the most severe extreme of depression, and dysthymia the lightest. Both respond especially well to therapy correcting thinking and behaviour – including the suggestions in this book – as well as therapy exploring their nature. They also respond to medication.

About 14-34% of people with substance abuse disorders have current depressive illness; 35-69% of these might have it for life. The following symptoms might occur only once in a lifetime or might be recurrent.

Symptoms. Two or more of the following 10 symptoms occur almost every day, when not due to a bereavement or conditions mentioned above: depressed mood most of the day; decreased interest/pleasure in almost all activities; significant weight loss when not dieting or weight gain (over 5% of body weight in a month) or decrease/increase in appetite; insomnia or hypersomnia; restlessness or lethargy; loss of energy; feelings of worthlessness or excessive or inappropriate guilt, not merely self-reproach; less ability to think or concentrate, or indecisiveness; recurrent thoughts of death, suicidal thoughts, suicide attempt; there has never been a manic, mixed or hypomanic episode (see bipolar disorders).

Dysthymia and major depression have similar symptoms, but they differ in onset, duration, persistence and severity. Major depressive episodes can be distinguished from someone's usual functioning but dysthymia has chronic, less severe symptoms which last for at least two years with less than two months' relief at a time.

Bipolar disorder. Also known as manic depression, this can involve a "manic" episode, a depressive episode or both cyclically. Onset usually occurs before age 30 but can be after 50. In most cases, the first episode involves a swing into the manic state. About 60% of people with a bipolar disorder meet criteria for chemical dependency, mainly alcohol.

"
It was explained to me that my 30 years of drinking had masked my manic depression. Psychiatrists told me that my adventurous and sometimes grandiose schemes – from organising street festivals and concerts to risking death in the Sahara – were an indication of a manic inclination. This was building when along came alcohol in considerable quantity. It was strong enough to suppress or distort the manic tendencies and at the same time increase the extent of any depressive periods.

I no longer drink alcohol. I follow a 12-Step programme. I also take non-addictive medication which is monitored with six-weekly blood tests. My life is manageable and I feel absolutely stabilised nowadays. **"**

Wylton
a dual-disorder recoverer

Wylton's story is similar to a few people I know in recovery with bipolar disorders. They have taken control of their lives to such an extent that, unless they speak of their condition, there is no way an onlooker could know they had a problem.

Symptoms for bipolar disorder, manic. There is a period of abnormally and persistently elevated, expansive or irritable mood, lasting at least one week.

During the mood disturbance, three or more of the following were present: inflated self-esteem or grandiosity, less need for sleep, more talkativeness, flight of ideas or feeling that thoughts are racing, distractibility to unimportant or irrelevant things, increase in goal-directed activity or psychomotor agitation, excessive involvement in pleasurable activities which could have painful consequences (eg, shopping sprees, sexual indiscretions, foolish business investments).

The mood swing caused marked impairment in occupational functioning, social activities or relationships, or necessitated hospitalisation.

People can be treated in either an addiction-treatment or mental-health setting, but the latter is more usual.

Schizophrenia. This is one of the most difficult dual diagnoses, but it is the degree to which a person has it which determines how successful treatment will be.

Symptoms include two or more of the following, each present for a significant part of a month – only one symptom is required if the delusions are bizarre or hallucinations consist of a voice with a running commentary or more than one voice: delusions, hallucinations, disorganised speech (derailment or incoherence), grossly disorganised or catatonic behaviour, negative symptoms. Social/occupational performance falls markedly. The disturbance persists for at least six months.

It is particularly important to consult dual-diagnosis experts because treatments for schizophrenia and for addiction often oppose each other. For example, it is recommended that addicts express their feelings but that is not recommended for shizophrenics. Addicts must be confronted about their addiction but it is not recommended that schizophrenics are confronted about their illness.

Having said that, family involvement helps both the ill member and the family to get help for themselves. Success with schizophrenia comes in small steps but it can come.

And remember: when schizophrenics stay away from drink and drugs, they have more control over any medication which helps them to lead lives with a greater semblance of normality.

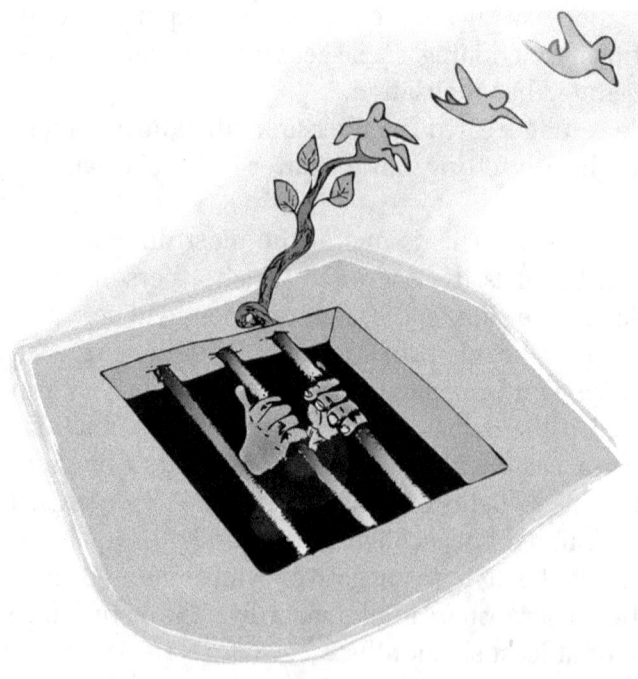

Anxiety disorders. These are the most common psychiatric problems in the general adult population.

When you feel in danger, the normal reaction is "fight or flight". Your brain tells your body to feel fear from the danger – your adrenal glands secrete stress hormones, your heart thumps faster, blood is pumped to your muscles which tense for action, and sweat cools your body – and urges you to take one solution or the other. If you react like this to a danger that does not exist, or if you restrict your activities to avoid having such a response, an anxiety or phobic disorder exists. Anxiety disorders include panic, phobic, obsessive-compulsive, post traumatic stress and generalised anxiety disorders.

Panic disorder is the most common among clients seeking addiction treatment, and occurs twice as often in female drug abusers as male drug abusers. One panic disorder, agoraphobia or fear of spaces, is the second-most common dual disorder among alcoholic women. Parents, children and siblings of clients with anxiety problems tend to share that anxiety problem.

The *DSM-IV* defines a panic attack as a period of intense fear or discomfort in which four or more of the following symptoms develop abruptly and reach a peak in 10 minutes: pounding or accelerated heart rate, sweating, trembling, sensations of shortness of breath or smothering, feeling of choking, chest pain/discomfort, nausea/abdominal distress, feeling dizzy/lightheaded/ faint, feelings of unreality/being detached from yourself, fear of losing control/going crazy, fear of dying, numbness or tingling, and chills or hot flushes.

Sufferers can get relief from proper breathing and relaxation techniques, a healthy diet which eliminates stimulants such as caffeine and nicotine, exercise to reduce muscle tension, and techniques to correct thoughts and beliefs – in other words, many of the recommendations in this book. Temporary medication might be needed.

Mental-health charity Mind offers advice on coping with a panic attack at: www.mind.org.uk/help/diagnoses_ and_conditions/panic_attacks

Phobic disorders are divided into social and specific phobias. The latter is an excessive or unreasonable persistent fear, triggered by the presence or anticipation of a specific object or situation. Examples are cats, spiders, flying, heights or receiving an injection. A social phobia is a persistent fear of social or performance situations in which you are exposed to unfamiliar people or possible scrutiny by others. You fear that you will act in a way which will be humiliating or embarrassing.

Both phobias can take the form of a panic attack. The avoidance or distress of the situation interferes with your normal routine, work or social activities or relationships, and/or there is distress about having the phobia. Fear of eating in public is not usually due to a phobia but to anorexia or bulimia.

People with social phobias are best treated first in individual, then in group, therapy. It is important to resolve the social phobia first, so that you do well in self-help programmes or other support groups.

Fear of social situations can be greatly reduced with training in good eye contact, posture, facial expression, voice quality and content and fluency of speech.

Mind offers more information on understanding phobias at www.mind.org.uk/help/diagnoses_and_conditions/phobias

Clinical anecdotes suggest that abuse of alcohol and minor tranquillisers is fairly common among people with obsessive-compulsive disorders.

Obsessions are persistent thoughts, impulses or images which are intrusive and cause anxiety. The most common are repeated thoughts about contamination (Howard Hughes is a famous example), repeated doubts (have I left the door unlocked?), a need to have things in a particular order, aggressive or horrific impulses (for example, to hurt your child or shout obscenities in church) and sexual imagery (recurrent pornography). These are unlikely to be related to a real-life problem.

Compulsions are other thoughts or actions which sufferers use to try to neutralise such thoughts and impulses. For example, if obsessed with contamination, you can compulsively hoover at midnight or scrub until the building stinks of ammonia. If you obsess about locking your front door, you try to neutralise the thoughts by compulsively checking to ensure that it is locked.

Obsessions or compulsions can displace useful and satisfying behaviour. Because they are distracting, they hamper cognitive tasks which need concentration, such as reading or computation. You might also avoid objects or situations which 'trigger' obsessions or compulsions.

This avoidance can severely restrict your life – for example, a mother who obsessed about shouting obscenities in church refused to attend her daughter's wedding.

People with OCD can benefit from behaviour and cognitive therapies, supported by medication. Reducing symptoms of this disorder reduces alcohol and drug intake, and *vice versa*. Again, Mind offers more details: www.mind.org.uk/help/diagnoses_and_conditions/ obsessive-compulsive_disorder.

Post traumatic stress disorder is something I have found to be common among people who have experienced abuse in childhood – which is most addictive people.

PTSD describes a range of psychological symptoms people can experience after a traumatic event, outside the normal human experience. The World Health Organisation has defined it as "a delayed or protracted response to a stressful event or situation (short or long-lasting) of an exceptionally threatening or long-lasting nature, which is likely to cause pervasive distress in almost anyone."

Many people contemplating coming into recovery will be familiar with the symptom of avoiding memories. This includes not only repressing memories (unable to remember aspects of the event) but also avoiding situations that remind you of the trauma, feeling detached/cut off and emotionally numb, being unable to express affection and that there is no point in planning for the future.

Symptoms tend to be dealt with when you come into

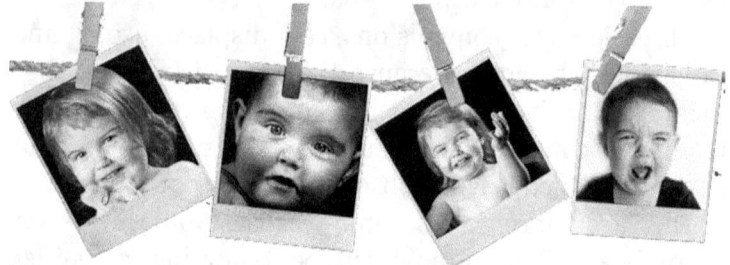

recovery, as you talk to your therapist about your childhood memories. These memories will surface only when you feel safe enough to allow them out, which is usually when you are comfortably into your drug-free recovery process.

You can read more information at www.mind.org.uk/help/diagnoses_and_conditions/post-traumatic_stress_disorder.

Below are the symptoms of borderline personality disorder according to 2009 government guidelines from the National Institute for Health and Clinical Excellence. A doctor will diagnose borderline personality disorder in people who have five or more of these symptoms and if the symptoms have a significant impact on them:

◊ having emotions that are up and down – for example, feeling confident one day and feeling despair another,

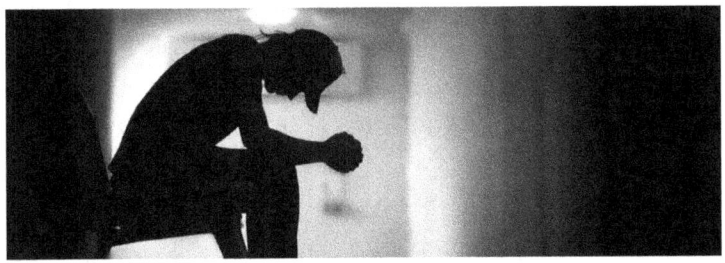

with feelings of emptiness and often anger

◊ difficulty in making and maintaining relationships
◊ an unstable sense of identity, thinking differently about yourself depending on who you are with
◊ taking risks or doing things without thinking about the consequences
◊ harming yourself or thinking about harming yourself – for example, cutting yourself or overdosing
◊ fearing being abandoned or rejected or being alone
◊ sometimes believing in things that are not real or true (delusions) or seeing or hearing things that are not really there (hallucinations).

Borderline personality disorder also tends to be simultaneously put in remission or dealt with as people talk to their therapists and follow a programme of recovery from addiction. More info: www.mind.org.uk/help/diagnoses_ and_conditions/borderline_personality_disorder

Antisocial personality disorder is thought to be the most common personality disorder co-existing with addiction, and is found more among men than women. This is known as 'psychopathy' under the *Mental Health Act 1983*.

It is a pattern of disregard for, and violation of, the rights of others. People with ASPD can perform acts which are grounds for arrest – although we can find them working among us also – fight, be deceitful and lack remorse for the effects of their actions on others. Boredom is a problem for people with ASPD and they can find it difficult to hold down a job for long or stay in a long-term relationship.

Many clients with APD can benefit from treatment, even if involuntary. The most effective therapy is to look at specific behaviours and ways of thinking rather than exploring the self.

Then there are people who have another type of "dual" diagnosis: a medical one rather than psychiatric – people with physical disabilities.

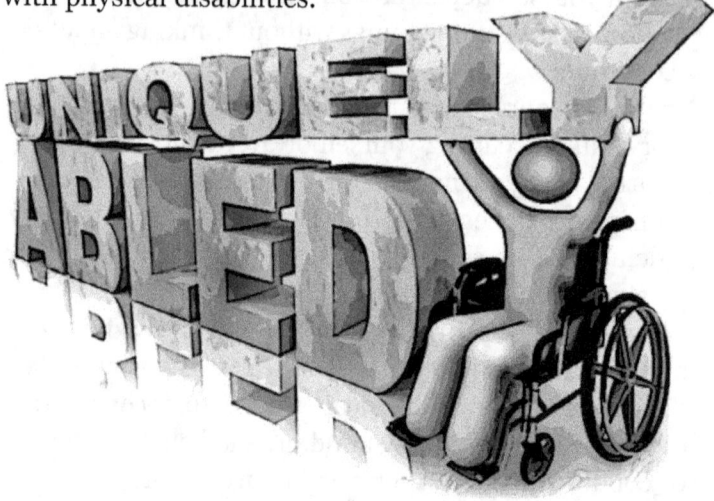

NOT A SPECIAL CASE: PEOPLE WITH
PHYSICAL DISABILITIES

Many people think that they must make allowances for people with physical disabilities who are addicted to drink, drugs or some other behaviour – but addiction is the most dangerous disability of them all. Indeed, the addiction might have led to the physical disability, through accident or illness, in the first place.

People can mistakenly spend time, energy and money treating symptoms rather than the addiction. This means little improvement for the disabled person and much stress for carers who can experience frustration, inadequacy, anger and physical and emotional exhaustion.

"Disability is commonly equated with illness, fostering the idea that disabled people are incapable of assuming responsibility for themselves, require repeated hospitalisations and must depend on mood-altering medication to function," state Dennis Straw and Sharon Schaschl, two of the authors of *Substance Abuse & Physical Disability* (edited by Allen W Heinemann) which remains the seminal book on this topic.

"Family, friends and the medical community often feel that there is little value for disabled people in achieving a chemically-free lifestyle. It is assumed that, without chemicals, they could not cope with what is perceived as a miserable existence," Schaschl and Straw note.

Some of their patients have received mood-altering medications since childhood and lived in protective environments which controlled their chemical use. When they left these environments and tried to integrate into an able-bodied society, increased chemical use became an equaliser. Addiction flourished.

Research on other patients, whose disabilities were the result of a later-onset trauma or illness, indicates that most were having problems related to mood-altering chemicals long before their disability.

Life problems experienced by people with disabilities – such as low self-esteem, poor hygiene, dependent lifestyle, lack of motivation, significant personality changes, memory deficits, depression, departure from personal values, isolation and unemployment – stem, as with all addicts, from the addiction and not from the physical disability. It cannot be made to be the excuse.

But change can be hard for carers, as permitting the addiction can ease their own uncomfortable feelings about the disability. Behaviours which are unacceptable in a non-disabled person might be permitted, ignored or excused in someone who has a disability.

Addiction might be encouraged as a means of socialising and achieving equality with able-bodied friends or as "one of my few pleasures". Carers might feel that they have no right to deny disabled people their choices, even if the choices are self-destructive. But enablers often lose sight of their own choices as they are manipulated to give permission or assistance to the disabled person to carry out destructive behaviour. The popular TV series *House* is an outstanding example of how this occurs.

As with all other addicts, mood-altering chemicals medicate feelings. But some feelings are a natural part of the grieving process; they must be experienced to accept disability as non-devaluing. Disabled people can appear to express their feelings, but the chemicals keep them dissociated from them.

What medications are non-damaging? These are viewed in two categories: convenience and essential, according to Straw and Schaschl. Addictive, mood-altering muscle relaxants to control muscle tension (spasticity) and narcotics to manage chronic pain are convenience medications. Anti-convulsants to control seizures are essential medications.

Mood-altering, addictive medications are inappropriate for chronic conditions. Antidepressants are appropriate when used with counselling and medical supervision.

Disabled people with chemical dependency must learn alternative ways to manage chronic pain, spasticity and stress. Relaxation, meditation, acupressure, biofeedback, self-hypnosis, diet, exercise, stretching, hot and cold packs, whirlpool and massage are effective replacement techniques. They can be developed independently or as part of a formal chronic-pain rehabilitation programme.

There seems to be about a three-month period after withdrawal of chemicals during which pain and spasticity seem intensified, as enough of our helpful brain chemicals have not yet been re-established and the nervous system adjusts to its unmedicated state.

Should someone be emotionally adjusted to his or her disability before entering treatment? Addiction stalls adjustment – addiction treatment accelerates it.

People with physical disabilities who have the courage to enter treatment might need help with writing materials/ tape recorders, architectural access and management of chronic pain and muscle tension. But otherwise they do not need special privileges.

Too often, disabled people have not been expected to take responsibility for themselves or their actions, and have learned to respond to the low expectations of others with self-pity, learned helplessness or manipulation. But acknowledging abilities allows disabled people to enjoy active and equal participation in recovery.

♥ ♥ ♥

12
Changing the future

If you have read this far — congratulations! It shows a great determination to succeed.

You have in your hands knowledge which, sadly, many generations before us did not. You cannot change past history but you can change future history – and not only your own. Your positive actions in recovery will affect everyone in your family who sees or knows about the difference. Your relationships will change for the better and be with people who are good for you. If you have children, you can give them a head start in life by handing down your new-found knowledge.

There are people in this world who have openly said that they would not have won their Oscars or Emmys without recovery and the support of their self-help fellowships. They have given positive messages to millions of people through their talent. There are others in recovery who teach, who are nurses and doctors, who help people through the legal system, who give employment, who bring up children, who reach into readers' lives through their writings... The list goes on.

People in recovery are a great and invaluable talent. The world is richer for having them. Welcome.

Deirdre

Further reading.

All the books mentioned in this book can be found at www.amazon.com or www.amazon.co.uk – simply enter the name and/or author in the website search box.

All the information mentioned as being available at www.addictiontoday.org is free of charge.

This includes a list of treatment centres and a list of self-help groups, all with contact details.